Monographs in Oral Science

Monographs in Oral Science

Vol. 17

Series Editor *G.M. Whitford*, Augusta, Ga.

KARGER Basel · Freiburg · Paris · London · New York · New Delhi · Bangkok · Singapore · Tokyo · Sydney

Assessment of Oral Health

Diagnostic Techniques and Validation Criteria

Volume Editor *R. V. Faller*, Mason, Ohio

81 figures, 17 in color, and 20 tables, 2000

KARGER

Basel · Freiburg · Paris · London · New York ·
New Delhi · Bangkok · Singapore · Tokyo · Sydney

••••••••••••••••••••••••••

R.V. Faller

The Procter & Gamble Company
Health Care Research Center
8700 Mason-Montgomery Road
Mason, OH 45040-9462

Library of Congress Cataloging-in-Publication Data

Assessment of oral health : diagnostic techniques and validation criteria / volume editor, R.V. Faller.
p. ; cm. – (Monographs in oral science, ISSN 0077-0892; vol. 17)
Includes bibliographical references and indexes.
ISBN 3805570309 (alk. paper)
1. Mouth – Diseases – Diagnosis. 2. Teeth – Diseases – Diagnosis. 3. Oral manifestations of general diseases. I. Faller, R.V. II. Series.
[DNLM: 1. Diagnosis, Oral – methods. 2. Mouth Diseases – diagnosis. 3. Tooth Diseases – diagnosis. WU 141 A846 2000]
RC815.A856 2000
616. 3′1075–dc21

00–038432

Drug Dosage. The authors and the publisher have exerted every effort to ensure that drug selection and dosage set forth in this text are in accord with current recommendations and practice at the time of publication. However, in view of ongoing research, changes in government regulations, and the constant flow of information relating to drug therapy and drug reactions, the reader is urged to check the package insert for each drug for any change in indications and dosage and for added warnings and precautions. This is particularly important when the recommended agent is a new and/or infrequently employed drug.

www.karger.com
Printed in Switzerland on acid-free paper by Reinhardt Druck, Basel
ISSN 0077–0892
ISBN 3–8055–7030–9

Contents

Preface

Over the past several years, a number of new methods have been developed for use in the diagnosis of oral disease states. Some of these methods may be applicable to dental practitioners and others may have greater applicability in a clinical situation. This volume of *Monographs in Oral Science* provides a description of a wide range of new oral diagnostic methods. A number of these methods are focused toward the specific assessment of disease states such as caries, calculus, plaque, gingivitis and periodontal disease. Other methods are more broad, focusing on methods to measure specific changes in oral morphology. Regardless of the method described, similarities exist when it comes to the validation of each method for general acceptance and use. Each method must be critically assessed in order to determine whether or not an appropriate validation has been done to confirm the robust nature of the technique or application.

The first eight chapters of this monograph provide descriptions of a range of new oral diagnostic techniques, the final chapter discusses considerations that must be taken into account regarding the validation requirements for each. While this monograph provides an overview of a series of specific new oral diagnostic methods, these are certainly not the only new methods under development for assessing oral disease states or morphology. Regardless of the technique being developed, the validation criteria laid out are applicable to any new oral diagnostic method.

R.V. Faller

Faller RV (ed): Assessment of Oral Health.
Monogr Oral Sci. Basel, Karger, 2000, vol 17, pp 1–19

Direct Digital Radiography for Caries Detection and Analysis

Mostafa Analoui, George K. Stookey

Indiana University School of Dentistry, Indianapolis, Ind., USA

Abstract

Recent developments in the field of electronic imaging have provided a new set of imaging tools for intra-oral imaging and clinical diagnosis. In this chapter, we review the general structure and characteristics of image sensors used in digital radiography and their application for clinical caries detection and analysis. An overview of the literature, comparing the diagnostic accuracy of digital and film-based radiography and the impact of image-processing methods, is provided. We also describe several approaches for quantitative assessment of radiographic images for caries detection and assessment. Examples include digital subtraction radiography, and 2-D and 3-D density profiling. To increase the accuracy and reduce observer variability the use of 3-D imaging and computer-aided diagnosis is presented as future direction for clinical caries diagnosis.

Introduction

The discovery of X-ray in 1895 was a historical step leading to the development of a broad class of diagnostic imaging methods commonly called 'radiography'. Shortly after its discovery, radiography found its application in dentistry in 1896 [1]. In the past 100 years, while maintaining the same principles of image formation, intra-oral radiography has made significant improvements [2]. These improvements include increased quality of X-ray production, understanding and reducing hazards associated with ionizing radiation and, more importantly, the constant evolution of radiographic image receptors. Throughout the first century of dental radiography, film has been the primary medium for radiographic imaging for both intra- and extra-oral applications. During this period, continuous developments in film technology focused on increasing film sensitivity and latitude, while reducing artifacts and processing time. Visual examination, often aided with various optical enhancements, constituted the primary mode of examination for radiographic images.

Introduction of digital computers in the early 1940s fueled a revolutionary chain of rapid developments in various fields of science, including the beginning steps in digital imaging for diagnostic applications. The computational power of digital computers, coupled with image and signal-processing algorithms, provided a wide range of options for image enhancement and analysis. The early approach for digital radiography involved scanning (digitizing) film-based radiographs into a computer, followed by image processing and display. This two-step process, also known as indirect digital radiography, gained significant popularity in research activities but not much use in clinical procedures. Moreover, such an indirectly formed digital image had, at best, the same information content as the film-based radiograph along with its characteristics and artifacts. The introduction of electronic image receptors in the late 1960s and their rapid improvements not only made the direct digital radiography (DDR) possible, but also led to the introduction of computed diagnostic imaging methods, such as computed tomography (CT).

The primary focus of this chapter is to review and assess the application of DDR for caries detection and analysis. The general characteristics of DDR systems will be discussed, followed by discussion of the attributes impacting their application in caries diagnosis. The impact of image enhancement methods on the visual examination of digital images, along with quantitative methods will be examined using some examples. This chapter will also offer a glimpse into future developments in imaging approaches for caries diagnosis.

Anatomy of a DDR System

Figure 1 shows a general block diagram depicting elements involved in a direct digital radiographic system. To better describe the functionality of each module in this diagram, the image acquisition ensemble is divided into three modules: (1) image receptor; (2) analog-to-digital converter (ADC), and (3) digital computer. Note that the ADC is typically integrated either within the sensor or in the computer. The combination of these three modules defines the difference between DDR and film-based radiography. The radiation reaching the surface of the image receptor is stored in an array of sensitive cells. The stored charge in each cell is then converted to a discrete level by ADC and transferred to the digital computer for storage, display and processing. Currently, there are two technologies in use for digital dental imaging.

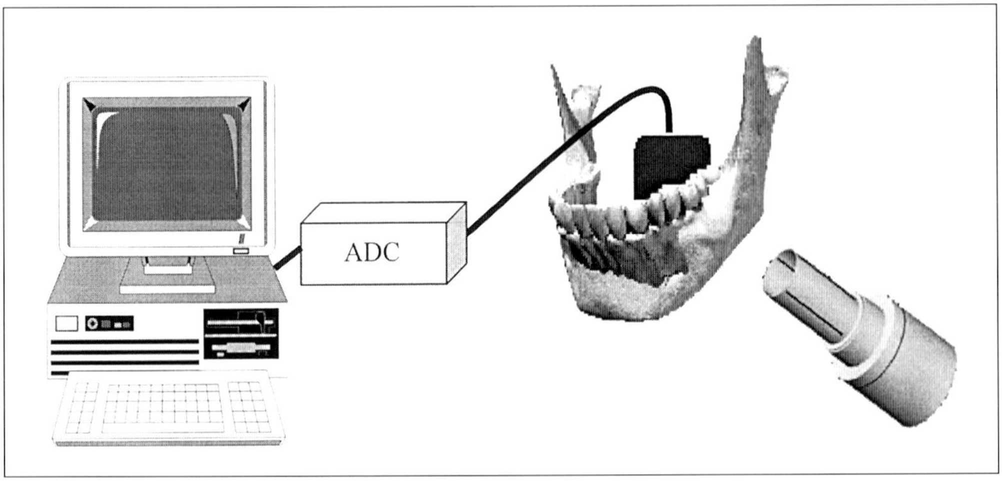

Fig. 1. A schematic diagram depicting elements involved in a direct digital radiographic (DDR) system. The diagram is intended to show the functional relationship between components and not clinical placement.

The first technology is composed of a group of digital image receptors that can transfer the captured image 'electronically' in real-time to the computer system. Charge-coupled device (CCD) technology is the first of the electronic receptors introduced in 1989 [3] for dental application. Currently, CCD-based receptors are the most common electronic receptors which have gone through significant improvements since their introduction. A CCD image receptor is composed of an array of individual small sensors, configured in a uniform and rectangular form. Each small sensor collects the X-ray energy imparted. The collection of these sensed signals will be transferred to the computer via the ADC unit to form the digital radiographic image. Active pixel sensor (APS) is another electronic image receptor [4] recently introduced and deployed in dental imaging, with promise of increased resolution, sensitivity, and enhanced system integration at a lower cost than CCD. An APS image receptor has a structure similar to the CCD receptor, except it offers direct access to each individual location within the sensor. This allows operation such as reading a small region of interest (ROI) or location-dependent processing of image on the chip.

Photostimulable storage phosphor (PSP) is the second category of imaging technology that has found some acceptance in dental radiography [5–7] and caries diagnosis [8–11]. PSP image receptors are fundamentally different from electronic receptors in terms of design and structure. PSP imaging requires a

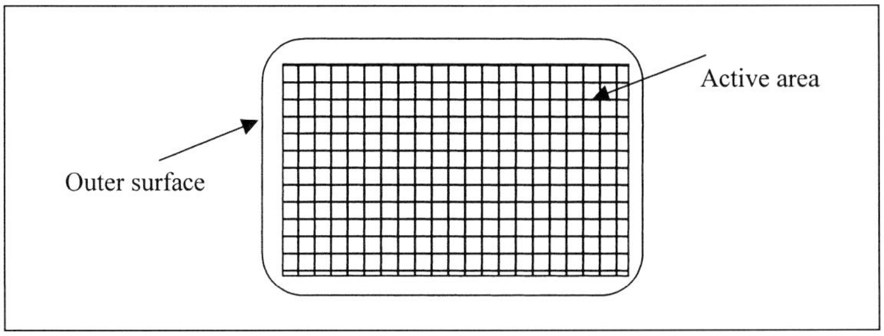

Fig. 2. Structure of an electronic image receptor.

scanning step and does not provide an immediate image. Despite the differences, PSP shares many of the characteristics of the electronic image receptor, which makes it an alternative approach for digital radiography.

Characteristics of Electronic Image Receptors

An electronic imager is composed of a discrete array of receptors uniformly distributed throughout its active area. Picture elements, also known as pixels (fig. 2), ideally act as independent receptors collecting the radiation received at the surface of the imager.[1] Each small square area in figure 2 represents 1 pixel. The charges collected by pixels are then converted to the discrete levels through ADC to form a digital image. These discrete levels correspond to optical densities developed at the film surface in film-based imaging.

Resolution

Since the resolution of an image receptor defines the size of a minimally detectable object, it is an extremely important characteristic for detection of lesions at an early stage of development, such as early caries diagnosis. The *theoretical* resolution of an electronic imager is defined by its pixel size. The resolution of DDR units currently available for dental applications ranges from 20 to 50 μm. Thus, at best such imaging systems can capture and render defects as small as 20 μm. Although film is an analog receptor, its resolution is limited by the size of silver halide and scattering within the film layers.

[1] The X-ray radiation is typically converted to visible photons through the scintillator layer covering the array of pixels.

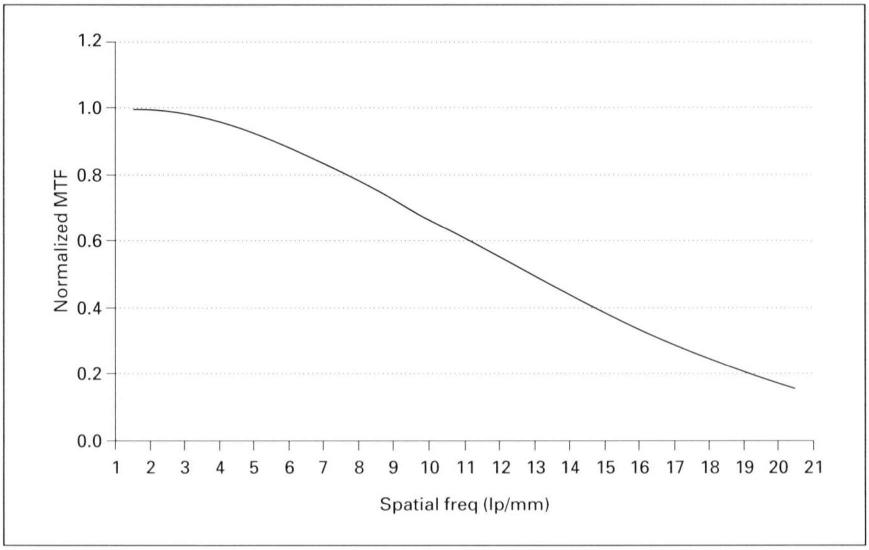

Fig. 3. MTF for a CCD-based image receptor with pixel size of 38 μm.

Dental radiographic films have been shown to have resolution between 14 and 20 line pairs (lp)/mm. This would be equivalent to a pixel size ranging from 25 to 36 μm.

Several design parameters limit the *effective* resolution of the image receptors significantly. Modulation transfer function (MTF) describes the resolving power of image receptors more accurately for a range of spatial frequencies [12]. Figure 3 shows the MTF for a CCD-based imager with a pixel size of 38 μm, which corresponds to approximately 13.3 lp/mm. Note that the spatial resolution of such a system is a decreasing function of spatial frequency.

Linearity

The sensitometric curve of radiographic film, describing the exposure vs. density, is known to have highly nonlinear behavior at the low and high end of the exposure scale [13]. This nonlinear response limits the dynamic range (latitude) of the film. More importantly, it complicates quantitative assessment of tissue density using densitometric approaches. CCD-based imagers inherently have an extremely linear exposure-count response throughout their dynamic range. Note that the count is typically converted and expressed by the gray level, which corresponds to optical density in the film-based approach.

Other Characteristics

Other characteristics of digital image receptors set them distinctly apart from film-based systems. Although these are important attributes of digital imagers, they will not have a direct impact on the accuracy of diagnosis. Among these attributes are: significant reduction of required exposure for formation of diagnostic image; consistent image quality (eliminating common errors associated with chemical processing and development), and instant image capture/display. Moreover, since the image is in the digital form, it can be duplicated (identical to the original image), stored and shared via electronic communication methods.

The following sections will overview various types of caries as well as the advantages and disadvantages of DDR systems for caries detection, along with a selective review of literature in this area.

Caries Classification According to Location

Dental caries is a pathologic process of localized loss of dental hard tissue by organic acid formation produced by the microbial deposits adhering to the tooth [1]. The gradual loss of dental hard tissue also modifies the structural characteristics of the tissue. Changes in the content and structure of dental tissue present a multitude of physical manifestations, which are commonly used for detection of disease. For example, visual examination relies on the difference between optical characteristics of sound and diseased enamel and dentine, while a tactile method primarily relies on structural changes within the tissue. Difference in absorption and scattering properties of healthy and diseased tissues is employed in the radiographic approach. This difference in mineral content is recorded by radiographic image receptors and depicted as optical density in film-based imaging or gray level in the digital radiographic approach.

The common radiographic sites for assessment of caries are interproximal, occlusal, smooth surfaces (buccal/lingual), pulpal, and root. Interproximal caries often forms a classic V-shaped radiolucent appearance, with the base of the lesion at the outer surface of the enamel and the tip pointing toward the dentinoenamel junction. Its severity is then classified based on its penetration within the enamel and dentine. Occlusal caries, the most prevalent location of caries, begins in the pits and fissures of the occlusal surfaces of the teeth. Radiographically the base of occlusal caries is at the dentinoenamel junction with its apex pointing toward the outer surface of the tooth, opposite to that of interproximal caries. Radiographic imaging of smooth surface caries is confounded by superimposition of layers of enamel and dentine. Unlike inter-

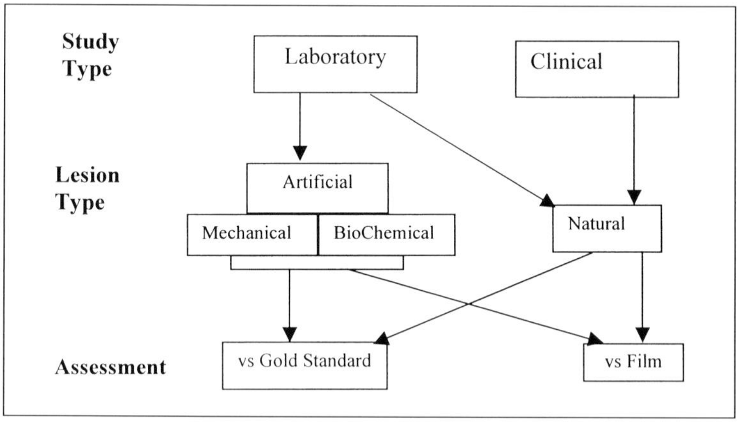

Fig. 4. Classification of approaches for evaluation of DDR for caries diagnosis.

proximal and occlusal caries, smooth surface caries appears on the radiograph as round radiolucent areas on the tooth surface. Root caries is commonly located on the interproximal cementoenamel junction with a saucer-shaped radiographic appearance [1]. In the following section we primarily focus on interproximal and occlusal caries.

Radiographic Caries Diagnosis Using DDR

With the introduction of any new diagnostic imaging approach, two critical questions are posed: (1) how does the new approach stack up against commonly accepted method(s), also known as conventional method(s), and (2) how does it match up against the gold standard(s). Answering these questions has primarily been the premise of several laboratory and clinical studies involving emerging imagers, such as xeroradiography, CCD, PSP, and APS. The diagram shown in figure 4 classifies study designs according to their hypotheses and objectives.

Although techniques such as xeroradiography [14, 15] and digitizing radiographs [16, 17] provided an early view into the use of digital imaging for caries diagnosis, this chapter focuses on more recent approaches based on direct digital imaging. Upon introduction of the first DDR system in dentistry, called radiovisiography (RVG) [3], several studies were designed to evaluate its diagnostic capability for various types of lesions. Wenzel et al. [18] compared the accuracy of conventional film radiographs, digitized radiographs, and

RVG for the detection of dentinal caries in occlusal surfaces of noncavitated extracted teeth. In this study 4 observers assessed 81 fully erupted extracted third molars using film-based radiography and DDR methods, followed by histological analysis to establish truth. Although processing of digitized and directly captured images tended to perform more accurately than conventional radiography, no statistically significant difference was observed. In a more comprehensive study Wenzel et al. [19] compared the diagnostic capability of CCD-based units (Trophy RVG, Sens-A-Ray, Visualix) and one PSP-based unit (Sordex Digora) for detection of occlusal caries. The study concluded that the four digital systems performed almost equally well for the detection of caries in vitro.

In a more recent study, White and Yoon [20] evaluated the performance of a digital CCD-based system (Schick CDR) for detecting proximal surface caries compared with film. Despite differences in sensitivity and specificity of each system, the overall results did not indicate any statistical difference.

It should be noted that studies involving mechanically created lesions have shown better performance for film than digital imagers [21, 22]. However, the above-mentioned reports along with several other studies [23–25] indicated comparable performance for digital imagers and film for detection of carious lesions based on the visual examination of radiographic images.

Impact of Image Post-Processing on Caries Diagnosis

Image processing offers a wide range of algorithms for image manipulation, which may impact the diagnostic utility of a given radiograph. Once a radiographic image is available in the digital form, regardless of being captured directly or digitized from film, all processing routines are applicable to it. Image enhancement algorithms, commonly employed in diagnostic imaging, offer a wide range of options for subjectively manipulating images to enhance their visual appearance.

Contrast/brightness manipulation, edge enhancement, histogram equalization, noise removal, and pseudocoloring [26] are among techniques commonly used for enhancing digital radiographic images. Several investigators have studied and reported the impact of such algorithms on caries diagnosis with a mixed outcome for their efficacy. Examples include the use of contrast enhancement for digitized and CCD images [18, 27] and edge enhancement [28], which have shown improvements in diagnosis of carious lesions as a result of enhancement. Other studies reported that techniques such as histogram equalization or reverse contrast [25] did not have any significant impact on the diagnostic quality of images for approximal caries.

Due to the subjectivity and task-dependence of image enhancement techniques one can expect that the mere use of such general techniques may not lead to an improvement in diagnosis, and perhaps can have a negative impact on diagnostic quality of images [27].

In general, the optimal image enhancement for a given diagnostic task is a function of: (a) imaging modality; (b) diagnostic task; (c) characteristic of display medium, and (d) human observer.

An effective and optimal image enhancement method should address the above parameters explicity.

General Issues for Evaluation of DDR Systems

Studies comparing DDR systems and film-based radiography typically include the following steps: (1) subject/specimen selection/preparation; (2) imaging the subjects/specimens using film and DDR techniques; (3) presenting the radiographic images to a group of examiners for visual examination, and (4) establishing ground truth on the existence and severity of lesions by the gold standard.

There are several confounding factors that adversely impact such a study design. For the sake of brevity this chapter focuses on step 3, i.e. image presentation and visual examination.

The first choice that must be made in this regard is the mode of image presentation: computer display vs. direct viewing of film on a viewing box. Digital images are intended to be displayed and viewed on the computer displays. However, in a comparative study the question is whether the film-based radiograph should be viewed using the conventional method (back-illuminated with the aid of a magnifying glass in a room with reduced illumination) or digitizing it and viewing it on the same monitor used for digital images. Clearly, each consideration has its own merit. Since resolution of common computer display devices is significantly less than film and digital imagers, displayed images appear much larger on the screen than the actual size of the objects. Moreover, the display devices have nonlinear characteristics that require calibration for a faithful and repeatable rendition of images. Also, the appearance of a displayed image is a function of preprocessing, color maps, and the software implementation. The standard presentation of diagnostic images on a calibrated display is of extreme importance, which is the subject of the evolving standards such as DICOM [29, 30].

The human factor is the other side of the coin in the visual examination of radiographic images. Radiologists, by training and experience, are more accustomed to read the radiographs using a conventional method of a viewing box, aided with a magnifying glass. To assure consistency and repeatability in the comparative study there is a need for uniform training for all examiners participating in such studies, along with sufficient experience in reading images on a computer display. In a longitudinal clinical study Eggertson et al. [31] showed that the intraexaminer agreement for a clinician with limited experience with digital radiographic images, but extensive experience in film-based radiography, increased from 0.36 to 0.75 and 0.61, respectively, while reading subsequent images.

The characteristics of a human visual system (HVS) is another important factor limiting the sensitivity of visual diagnosis, especially for the detection of carious lesions. It is known that HVS can differentiate a limited number of gray levels in a noncontrasted viewing approach. In a study based on the visual assessment of 10 dentists, including 6 oral radiologists, Ohki et al. [28] reported that 32 levels of gray levels would be acceptable for detection of interproximal caries. Comparing this level of visual sensitivity to the content of radiographic images, about 1,000 gray levels in film and 256 gray levels for images displayed on nonmedical grade monitors, it is quite possible for a human observer to overlook minute variations and changes in the image density. Moreover, common digital image receptors have dynamic ranges in excess of 4,096 gray levels. However, since the common computer monitors display only up to 256 gray levels and significant cost is associated with monitors with higher depth monitors, all DDR manufacturers limit the captured information to 256 gray levels. These visual and display limitations necessitate employing more objective and quantitative approaches.

Quantitative Radiographic Approach

Perhaps quantitative radiographic assessment is the strongest aspect of digital diagnostic imaging. The common attributes analyzed and measured in nontime-varying quantitative methods can be classified into one of two categories: (1) geometric, and (2) densitometric parameters. Geometric information includes parameters such as length, angle, area and volume of normal and abnormal anatomy. Densitometric information mainly concerns tissue mass and density as they appear on the radiograph.

Digital subtraction (DS) is the common method for detecting differences in two or more images of the same anatomical site [32, 33]. In this approach, the images under study are subtracted mathematically. Wherever the images have identical content the subtraction image contains zero values. The areas with different gray levels will lead to non-zero values in the subtraction image.[2] There are two basic assumptions made prior to subtracting images, i.e. the images are captured under the same imaging geometry and exposures [34, 35]. Despite various approaches for minimizing exposure and geometric errors in the clinical application there is a chance for violation of these assumptions. To minimize the errors associated with exposure variation one has to take appropriate measures during image capture and chemical development steps. These measures include consistency in X-ray machine setup (kVp, mA, time, collimation) and chemical development (for film-based imaging). To further reduce errors due to exposure inconsistencies, various imaging algorithms have been proposed for post-processing. Examples include the use of standard reference phantoms and anatomical landmarks [36–38].

To control the geometric setting of imaging in a clinical situation, film- and sensor-holding devices, along with custom-made bite registration, are commonly used. To increase the accuracy of patient positioning, Hausmann et al. [39] devised a stereo video-based technique which showed significant improvement in reproducibility through a complicated and expensive setup. Computer-based approaches based on projectionally invariant structures were also proposed and tested to further reduce geometric errors [40].

Most studies reporting the use of DS in caries diagnosis have tested this method in vitro for film-based radiography. Maggio et al. [41] used a standardized imaging geometry to image the development of caries in a time-lapsed film-based radiography. The primary objective of this work was to evaluate a model for dentinal caries progression. To assess the impact of DS for detection of secondary caries, Nummikoski et al. [42] studied defects created mechanically. This study reported that subtraction radiography was superior to conventional radiography in recurrent caries detection, mainly by reducing the false-positive diagnoses. In a similar study, Wenzel and Halse [43] used 38 fully erupted, extracted third molars without clinical cavitation in the occlusal surface. A radiograph was made of each tooth before and after 5, 10, and 20 min of stannous fluoride treatment. Two observers assessed the stannous fluoride-treated radiograph and the subtraction images on a monitor, and no significant differences were reported.

Generally, studies using lesions of large extent [44] did not report a significant difference between DS and conventional radiography. One can postulate that due to the large extent of lesions in these cases, the advantage of DS is not appropriately deployed. Hence, there is a need for testing the DS approach

[2] Note that gray levels in subtraction images are typically mapped and scaled such that they can be displayed on a computer display.

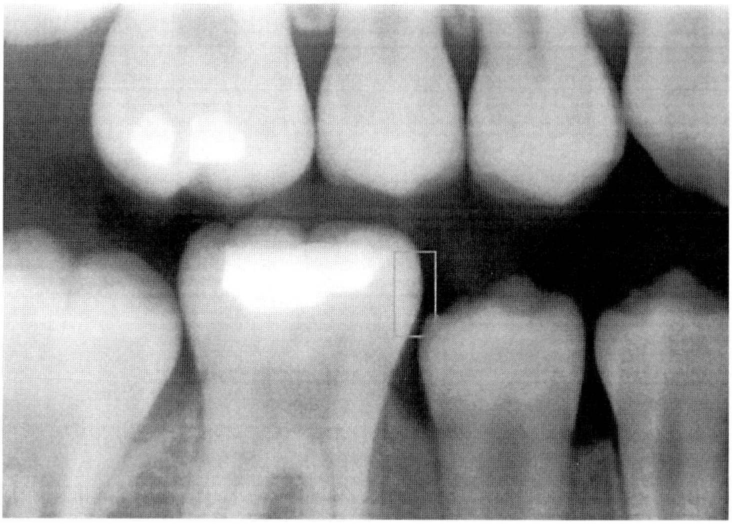

Fig. 5. A digital radiograph captured at 12 bbp in a clinical study. The rectangular ROI is further investigated through line and area profiling.

for interproximal and occlusal caries at an early stage of development. Such studies need to consider the impact of DS in visual detection as well as quantification of lesion severity.

Since DS requires at least two images for subtraction, it is commonly used for longitudinal assessment of lesion progress/regression. However, it is possible to assess the status of caries quantitatively using a single set of radiographs. One approach would be use of reference phantom objects of known density. An aluminum stepwedge is a common reference object used for densitometric assessment of lesions [45, 46]. The reference object provides two specific benefits: (1) contrast correction, and (2) quantitative measurement. Due to difficulties in the clinical use of such reference objects and variation in the superimposing soft tissue, a profiling approach can be considered as an alternative.

In the profiling method, line and area density profiles are computed for a ROI. In this approach the reference sound tissues are selected within the same image, hence it is appropriate mainly for within-patient quantitative comparisons. Figure 5 shows an in vivo digital radiograph captured using a 12-bit CCD imager and a 70-kVp X-ray generator. ROI marks a rectangular area on the approximal site of the first permanent mandibular molar.

Figure 6a shows the magnified ROI and six horizontal profile lines superimposed on the image. The density along each line is plotted in figure 6b.

Profiles are aligned such that the outer edge of the enamel is represented by pixel 0 on the horizontal axes of the plot. In an ideal radiographic image, one may expect a sudden drop in the gray level at the transition from enamel to background (soft tissue). However, because of the gradual decrease in enamel thickness, curvature of the approximal surface, finite resolution of the imager, and beam scattering, even sound enamel shows a gradual decrease in gray levels traversing the profile from enamel to background. A lesioned area shows a similar response but the line density profile decline starts earlier and continues faster than the line profile of sound enamel. In this example, the blue profile (the third profile from the top in the image) shows the deepest part of the lesion.

A similar approach can be used to profile the entire ROI as a single area. Such an approach will create area profiles typically depicted as surface plots. Figure 7 shows the area of profile for the ROI marked in figure 6a. Note that the lesioned area is depicted as a groove surrounded by enamel. Area profiles can be used to assess lesion depth and estimate mineral loss.

Beyond Basics: Computer-Aided Detection and 3-D Imaging

This section briefly covers two evolving areas in radiographic caries diagnosis, i.e. automatic caries detection and 3-D imaging. The introduction of DDR systems has been instrumental for increased activities in these areas.

Among several sources of variability, such as beam quality, receptor types, projection geometry, and observers, studies have found the largest source of variation to be the observer [47]. This issue along with a weak correlation between clinical appearance and radiographic findings [48], has sparked a new interest in computer-aided detection and analysis (CADA) of carious lesions.

Detection of lesions in the CADA approach is based on computer models describing the radiographic characteristics and appearance of carious lesions. Such models describe the sound and carious lesions in a rule-based approach or through statistical models. Examples of such approaches include the early work of Pitts [49] and Pitts and Renson [50], who reported significant improvement in the reproducibility of the detection process. In a different approach, Heaven et al. [51] reported that a CADA-based approach performed better than clinical examiners in vitro using simulated carious lesions. Another example of such an approach, developed by Logicon Inc., is based on a neural network model specifically trained for detection of interproximal caries.

Development of such approaches is greatly needed, as the focus is turning toward detection of lesions at very early stages. It is also important to assess the performance of the CADA-based approach in a clinical setting for such lesions.

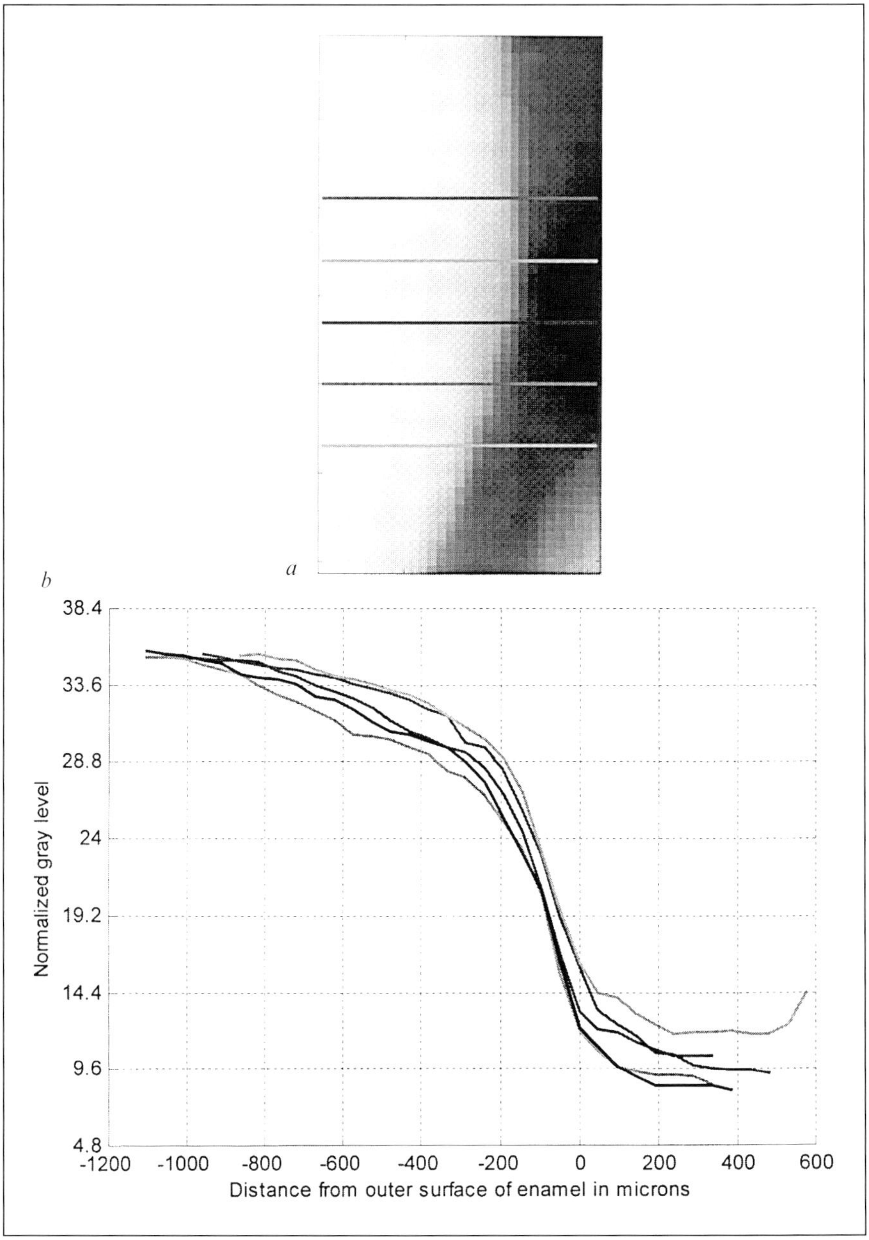

Fig. 6. a Rectangular ROI selected from figure 5. *b* Profiles along the lines shown in *a*. All profile lines are aligned such that the outer enamel edge corresponds to the zero value on the horizontal axis. Positive and negative numbers indicate the distance from the outer enamel edge, outside and inside enamel, respectively.

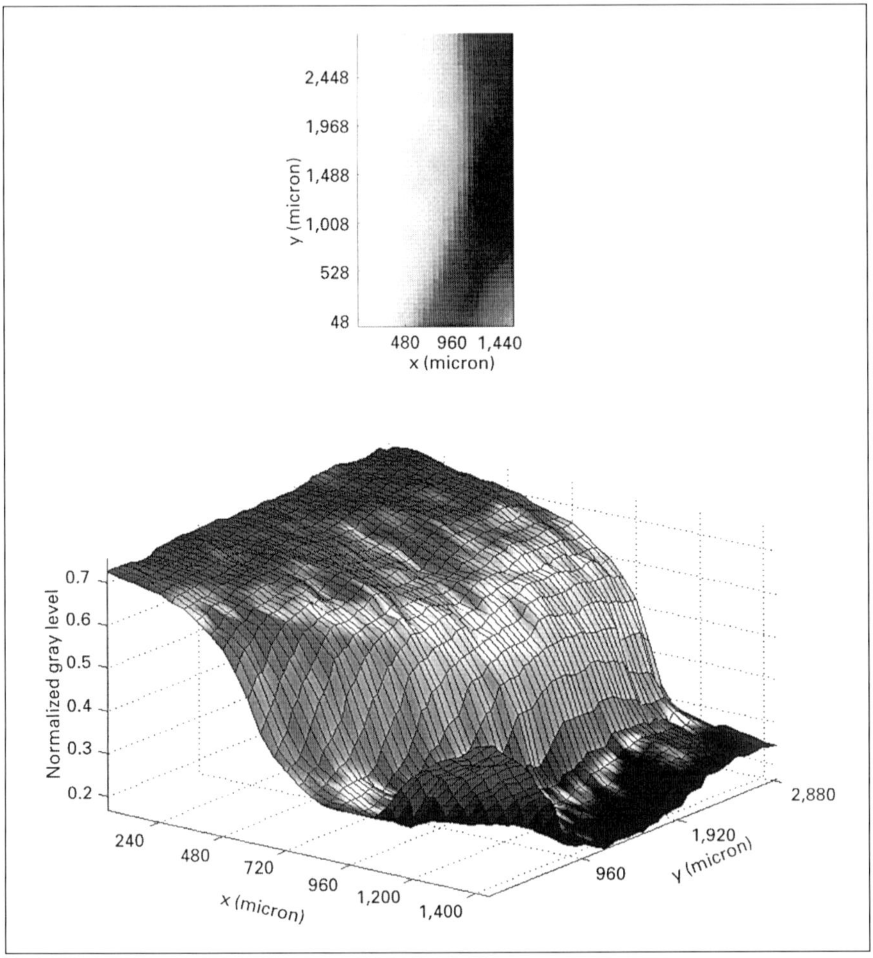

Fig. 7. Surface plot for ROI shown on the top. The plateau at higher level defines the sound enamel and grooves within this plateau show the extent and severity of mineral loss within that area.

Since the anatomy and tissues under study are defined by 3-D structures, it seems natural to expect improvement in diagnosis if the 3-D images of the tissues and anatomical sites were available. Traditionally, clinical 3-D imaging tended to be expensive with low resolution. Recent advances in computed imaging have reduced the cost of 3-D imaging, while increasing the resolution. However, the cost associated with these approaches still is not jusitifiable for routine caries diagnosis. Tuned aperture CT (TACT) is among the emerging

3-D imaging techniques that have shown promising results for various imaging tasks in dentistry. A recent in vitro evaluation of TACT for detection of interproximal and occlusal lesion [52] showed that TACT performed comparable to film-based radiography. Although TACT is not designed primarily for caries diagnosis, it is expected that deployment of such systems in the dental diagnosis may have significant impact on detection and assessment for dental caries.

Concluding Remarks

The introduction of new digital imaging receptors has sparked a great deal of interest in the evaluation of their performance for caries diagnosis. Since most reported studies have indicated no statistical difference between film and digital receptors for caries diagnosis, it is time to move beyond the comparison stage and focus on utilizing the unique characteristic of the digital receptors. Considering linearity, consistency in image quality, improvements in resolution and dynamic range, and instant image capture of electronic imagers, increased activities are expected in the following three areas for caries diagnosis.

(1) Clinical quantitative approaches to detect proximal and occlused carious lesions and monitor their progress/regressions. Quantitative approaches enable the discovery of demineralized areas much smaller than those commonly detected by visual examination of radiographic images. Such an early detection may provide a better chance for reversing the course of demineralization, hence reducing the need for restorative treatment.

(2) The development of sophisticated imaging algorithms for the automatic detection of carious lesions seems to have potential for aiding clinicians by increasing diagnostic accuracy. As digital imaging systems gain more acceptance in dental offices, and caries detection routines are made more accurate and easier to use, it is expected that more effort in using such methods for clinical diagnosis will be seen.

(3) Although clinical use of 3-D imaging for caries diagnosis seems to be far-fetched and not justifiable in terms of cost and complexity at this time, future reductions in cost and clinical application of such approaches in dentistry will provide a more accurate and realistic view of carious lesions.

References

1 Langland OE, Langlais RP: Principles of Dental Imaging. Baltimore, Williams & Wilkins, 1997.
2 Pitts NB: The use of bitewing radiographs in the management of dental caries: Scientific and practical considerations. Dentomaxillofac Radiol 1996;25:5–16.
3 Mouyen F, Benz C, Sonnabend E, Lodter JP: Presentation and physical evaluation of RadioVisioGraphy. Oral Surg Oral Med Oral Pathol 1989;68:238–242.
4 Cavadore C, Solhusvik J, Magnan P, Gautrand A, Degerli Y, Lavernhe F, Farre JA, Saint-Pe O, Davancens R, Tulet M: Design and characterization of CMOS imagers with two different technologies; in Blouke MM (ed): Proc SPIE. Solid State Sensor Arrays: Development and Applications II. 1998, vol 3301, pp 140–150.
5 Conover GL, Hildebolt CF, Yokoyama-Crothers N: Comparison of linear measurements made from storage phosphor and dental radiographs. Dentomaxillofac Radiol 1996;25:268–273.
6 Hildebolt CF, Fletcher G, Yokoyama-Crothers N, Conover GL, Vannier MW: A comparison of the response of storage phosphor and film radiography to small variations in X-ray exposure. Dentomaxillofac Radiol 1997;26:147–151.
7 Huda W, Rill LN, Benn DK, Pettigrew JC: Comparison of a photostimulable phosphor system with film for dental radiology. Oral Surg Oral Med Oral Pathol Oral Radiol Endod 1997;83:725–731.
8 Moystad A, Svanaes DB, Risnes S, Larheim TA, Grondahl HG: Detection of approximal caries with a storage phosphor system. A comparison of enhanced digital images with dental X-ray film. Dentomaxillofac Radiol 1996;25:202–206.
9 Nielsen LL, Hoernoe M, Wenzel A: Radiographic detection of cavitation in approximal surfaces of primary teeth using a digital storage phosphor system and conventional film, and the relationship between cavitation and radiographic lesion depth: An in vitro study. Int J Paediatr Dent 1996;6: 167–172.
10 Svanaes DB, Moystad A, Risnes S, Larheim TA, Grondahl HG: Intraoral storage phosphor radiography for approximal caries detection and effect of image magnification: Comparison with conventional radiography. Oral Surg Oral Med Oral Pathol Oral Radiol Endod 1996;82:94–100.
11 Versteeg KH, Sanderink GC, Velders XL, van Ginkel FC, van der Stelt PF: In vivo study of approximal caries depth on storage phosphor plate images compared with dental X-ray film. Oral Surg Oral Med Oral Pathol Oral Radiol Endod 1997;84:210–213.
12 Giger ML, Doi K: Investigation of basic imaging properties in digital radiography. I. Modulation transfer function. Med Phys 1984;11:287–295.
13 Thompson MA, Hattaway MP, Hall JD, Dowd SB: Principles of Imaging Science and Protection. Philadelphia, Saunders, 1997.
14 White SC, Gratt BM: Clinical trials of intraoral dental xeroradiography. J Am Dent Assoc 1979; 99:810–816.
15 White SC, Gratt BM, Bauer JG: A clinical comparison of xeroradiography and film radiography for the detection of proximal caries. Oral Surg Oral Med Oral Pathol 1988;65:242–248.
16 Kassebaum DK, McDavid WD, Dove SB, Waggener RG: Spatial resolution requirements for digitizing dental radiographs. Oral Surg Oral Med Oral Pathol 1989;67:760–769.
17 Wenzel A, Fejersko O, Kidd E, Joyston-Bechal S, Groeneveld A: Depth of occlusal caries assessed clinically, by conventional film radiographs, and by digitized, processed radiographs. Caries Res 1990;24:327–333.
18 Wenzel A, Hintze H, Mikkelsen L, Mouyen F: Radiographic detection of occlusal caries in noncavitated teeth. A comparison of conventional film radiographs, digitized film radiographs, and RadioVisioGraphy. Oral Surg Oral Med Oral Pathol 1991;72:621–626.
19 Wenzel A, Borg E, Hintze H, Grondahl HG: Accuracy of caries diagnosis in digital images from charge-coupled device and storage phosphor systems: An in vitro study. Dentomaxillofac Radiol 1995;24:250–254.
20 White SC, Yoon DC: Comparative performance of digital and conventional images for detecting proximal surface caries. Dentomaxillofac Radiol 1997;26:32–38.
21 Dagenais ME, Clark BG: Receiver operating characteristics of RadioVisioGraphy. Oral Surg Oral Med Oral Pathol Oral Radiol Endod 1995;79:238–245.

22 Parks ET, Miles DA, Van Dis ML, Williamson GF, Razmus TF, Bricker SL: Effects of filtration, collimation, and target-receptor distance on artificial approximal enamel lesion detection with the use of RadioVisioGraphy. Oral Surg Oral Med Oral Pathol 1994;77:419–426.
23 Hintze H, Wenzel A, Jones C: In vitro comparison of D- and E-speed film radiography, RVG, and visualix digital radiography for the detection of enamel approximal and dentinal occlusal caries lesions. Caries Res 1994;28:363–367.
24 Russell M, Pitts NB: Radiovisiographic diagnosis of dental caries: Initial comparison of basic mode videoprints with bitewing radiography. Caries Res 1993;27:65–70.
25 Dove SB, McDavid WD: A comparison of conventional intra-oral radiography and computer imaging techniques for the detection of proximal surface dental caries. Dentomaxillofac Radiol 1992;21:127–134.
26 Gonzalez RC, Wintz P: Digital Image Processing. Addison-Wesley, 1992.
27 Shrout MK, Russell CM, Potter BJ, Powell BJ, Hildeboldt CF: Digital enhancement of radiographs: Can it improve caries diagnosis? J Am Dent Assoc 1996;127:469–473.
28 Ohki M, Okano T, Nakamura T: Factors determining the diagnostic accuracy of digitized conventional intraoral radiographs. Dentomaxillofac Radiol 1994;23:77–82.
29 Bidgood WDJ, Horii SC: Modular extension of the ACR-NEMA DICOM standard to support new diagnostic imaging modalities and services. J Digit Imaging 1996;9:67–77.
30 Blume H, Hemminger BM: Image presentation in digital radiology: Perspectives on the emerging DICOM display function standard and its application. Radiographics 1997;17:769–777.
31 Eggertson H, Analoui M, Isaacs RL, Eckert G, Stookey GK: Longitudinal approximal caries detection using digital radiographic images. Caries Res 1998;32:293–293
32 Bragger U, Burgin W, Lang NP, Buser D: Digital subtraction radiography for the assessment of changes in peri-implant bone density. Int Oral Maxillofac Implants 1991;6:160–166.
33 Jeffcoat MK, Reddy MS, van den Berg HR, Bertens E: Quantitative digital subtraction radiography for the assessment of peri-implant bone change. Clin Oral Implants Res 1992;3:22–27.
34 Janssen PT, van Palenstein H, van Aken J: The effect of in-vivo-occurring errors in the reproducibility of radiographs on the use of the subtraction technique. J Clin Periodontol 1989;16: 53–58.
35 Webber RL, Ruttimann UE, Heaven TJ: Calibration errors in digital subtraction radiography. J Periodontal Res 1990;25:268–275.
36 Ohki M, Okano T, Yamada N: A contrast-correction method for digital subtraction radiography. J Periodontal Res 1988;23:277–280.
37 Ruttimann UE, Webber RL, Schmidt E: A robust digital method for film contrast correction in subtraction radiography. J Periodontal Res 1986;21:486–495.
38 Analoui M, Roberts WE: Radiographic contrast correction for quantitative analysis of bone adaptation ahead of a moving tooth; in Davidovitch Z (ed): Biological Mechanisms of Tooth Movement and Craniofacial Adaptation. 1996, pp 481–490.
39 Hausmann E, Allen K, Loza J, Buchanan W, Cavanaugh PF Jr: Validation of quantitative digital subtraction radiography using the electronically guided alignment device/impression technique. J Periodontol 1996;67:895–899.
40 Dunn SM, van der Stelt PF, Ponce A, Fenesy K, Shah S: A comparison of two registration techniques for digital subtraction radiography. Dentomaxillofac Radiol 1993;22:77–80.
41 Maggio JJ, Hausmann EM, Allen K, Potts TV: A model for dentinal caries progression by digital subtraction radiography. J Prosthet Dent 1990;64:727–732.
42 Nummikoski PV, Martinez TS, Matteson SR, McDavid WD, Dove SB: Digital subtraction radiography in artificial recurrent caries detection. Dentomaxillofac Radiol 1992;21:59–64.
43 Wenzel A, Halse A: Digital subtraction radiography after stannous fluoride treatment for occlusal caries diagnosis. Oral Surg Oral Med Oral Pathol 1992;74:824–828.
44 Bragger U, Burgin W, Marconi M, Hasler RU, Lang NP: Influence of contrast enhancement and pseudocolar transformation on the diagnosis with digital subtraction images (DSI) J Periodontal Res 1994;29:95–102.
45 Pitts NB: Detection and measurement of approximal radiolucencies by computer-aided image analysis. Oral Surg Oral Med Oral Pathol 1984;58:358–366.

46 Allen KM, Hausmann E: Analytical methodology in quantitative digital subtraction radiography: Analysis of the aluminum reference wedge. J Periodontol 1996;67:1317–1321.
47 Mera T, Okano T, Ishikawa I: Alveolar bone changes after initial preparation observed by subtraction radiography (in Japanese). Nippon Shishubyo Gakkai Kaishi 1985;27:902–911.
48 Rugg-Gunn AJ, Holloway PJ, Davies TG: Partial recording in caries incremental studies in English schoolchildren. Community Dent Oral Epidemiol 1975;3:11–19.
49 Pitts NB: Systems for grading approximal carious lesions and overlaps diagnosed from bitewing radiographs. Proposals for future standardization. Community Dent Oral Epidemiol 1984;12:114–122.
50 Pitts NB, Renson CE: Reproducibility of computer-aided image-analysis-derived estimates of the depth and area of radiolucencies in approximal enamel. J Dent Res 1985;64:1221–1224.
51 Heaven TJ, Weems RA, Firestone AR: The use of a computer-based image analysis program for the diagnosis of approximal caries from bitewing radiographs. Caries Res 1994;28:55–58.
52 Tyndall DA, Clifton TL, Webber RL, Ludlow JB, Horton RA: TACT imaging of primary caries. Oral Surg Oral Med Oral Pathol Oral Radiol Endod 1997;84:214–225.

Mostafa Analoui, PhD, School of Dentistry, Indiana University,
1121 West Michigan Street, Indianapolis, IN 46202 (USA)
Tel. +1 317 274 5250, Fax +1 317 278 3018, E-Mail manaloui@iupui.edu

Faller RV (ed): Assessment of Oral Health.
Monogr Oral Sci. Basel, Karger, 2000, vol 17, pp 20–31

Relationship of Surface Epithelium Concentrations of IL-1α and IL-1β to Clinical Inflammation during Experimental Gingivitis

Aaron Biesbrock, Chyon Hwa Yeh

The Procter & Gamble Company, Cincinnati, Ohio., USA

Abstract

Experimental evidence has clearly demonstrated that IL-1 cytokine levels increase in experimental gingivitis (EG) models in response to plaque accumulation following the cessation of oral hygiene. These changes in cytokine production are reported to occur prior to visible signs of clinical inflammation, and as such may represent early markers of gingival inflammation. This clinical study used a novel dermal sampling tape as a method to collect cytokines from gingival epithelium, as opposed to the more commonly sampled gingival crevicular fluid. The primary objective of the study was to examine the relationship between changes in cytokine levels and clinical inflammation. Ten subjects participated in a 14-day EG model, where 5 days following a dental prophylaxis subjects refrained from all oral hygiene measures for 14-days. Clinical measures including the Löe-Silness Gingival Index (GI), a bleeding index derived from the GI, and the inflammation index (II) were made at baseline prior to the initiation of the EG period and following 14 days of EG. Dermal tape samples were collected from the right posterior buccal quadrant of each subject at both baseline and day 14. The tapes were extracted and the extracts analyzed for both IL-1α and IL-1β by ELISA. Results of this study indicate that over a 14-day EG period statistically significant ($p < 0.05$) increases in GI, gingival bleeding, II, and IL-1α were observed (tested by matched-pairs t test and Wilcoxon signed ranks test). A directional increase in IL-1β was also observed. Linear regression analyses demonstrated a strong positive correlation between the number of gingival bleeding sites from the region of gingiva sampled with Sebutape® and IL-1α ($r = 0.93$), as well as IL-1β ($r = 0.90$). In addition, linear regression analyses also demonstrated a strong positive correlation between the mean II score from the region of gingiva sampled with Sebutape® and IL-1α ($r = 0.93$), as well as IL-1β ($r = 0.86$). Similar correlations were observed for whole mouth scores of the number of gingival bleeding sites and mean II with respect to IL-1α and IL-1β levels. Collectively, these data confirm the utility of the dermal tape for sampling epithelium cytokine levels from the gingiva and demonstrate a strong positive correlation between IL-1α and IL-1β concentrations and gingival inflammation.

Introduction

Interleukin 1 (IL-1) is one of the primary mediators of the initial human host response to microbial challenge and plays a multifunctional role in the initiation and propagation of the host inflammatory response [1]. IL-1 is produced as two structurally related but distinct proteins, IL-1α and IL-1β [2, 3]. IL-1α and IL-1β manifest similar pro-inflammatory properties, although IL-1β is reported to be more potent [4, 5]. The reported pro-inflammatory properties of IL-1 include inhibition of bone formation, enhancement of bone resorption, stimulation of prostaglandin and thromboxane synthesis, stimulation of collagenase and protease production, potentiation of neutrophil degranulation and superoxide production, enhancement of endothelial cell leukocyte adhesion, and stimulation of fibroblast and keratinocyte proliferation [5–11]. While macrophages and monocytes are the most potent producers of IL-1, other cell types such as neutrophils, fibroblasts, Langerhans cells, and keratinocytes have also been shown to produce IL-1 [2, 12–15]. IL-1 expression is inducible, during inflammation, injury, immunologic challenge, or infection, as unstimulated cells have been shown to have minimal basal levels [2]. Interestingly, IL-1α expression appears to be constitutive in keratinocytes as high basal levels are detectable in unstimulated cells [16, 17].

The clinical ramifications of complete cessation of oral hygiene practices in humans includes the accumulation of bacterial plaque and the development of gingivitis characterized by marked gingival inflammation and bleeding [18, 19]. In experimental gingivitis models where gingivitis is deliberately induced by the cessation of oral hygiene, concentrations of IL-1 have been shown to increase sharply within the first week of no hygiene [20, 21]. Furthermore, IL-1 has been reported to increase prior to visible signs of clinical inflammation [21, 22]. These studies have focused on sampling gingival crevicular fluid (GCF), a serum transudate/exudate derived from capillary beds underlying the junctional epithelium in the gingival crevice. Sampling of GCF from the gingival crevice is accomplished by placing a strip of filter paper in the crevice [23]. Recently, a dermal sampling tape has become commercially available, which offers an alternative method for sampling cytokines from a defined area of epithelium [24, 25]. The objective of this study was to explore the utility of Sebutape® in sampling oral epithelium for cytokine levels, as well as to examine the relationship of surface epithelium concentrations of IL-1α and IL-1β to alterations in clinical inflammation and gingival bleeding.

Study Design and Methods

The study consisted of three periods involving 10 subjects. Change in gingival inflammation was induced through the addition and removal of oral hygiene across study periods. Clinical gingival inflammation (gingivitis) was assessed by modified Löe-Silness Gingival Index (GI) and by the inflammation index (II) [26, 27]. At screening, a total of 30 subjects were examined for bleeding following gingival margin stimulation with a UNC-15 periodontal probe. Subjects were rank-ordered by the number of bleeding sites and the 8 subjects with the highest number, as well as the 2 subjects with the lowest number were enrolled in the study.

During period 1, subjects were examined by an examiner who employed the GI and a second examiner who employed the II. The subjects rinsed thoroughly with tap water following each examination. A dental scaling/prophy was conducted on these subjects within 2 days of their period-1 assessment. No attempt was made to modify oral hygiene habits.

Five days following the prophies, subjects were seen for period 2. Subjects were again examined by an examiner who employed the GI and a second examiner who employed the II. The following day Sebutape® samples were collected from the right posterior buccal maxillary quadrant. At this point the subjects were instructed to cease all oral hygiene practices (brushing, flossing and rinsing) for 14 days.

Fourteen days following the cessation of oral hygiene, subjects were seen for period 3. The clinical examinations were repeated as in periods 1 and 2. The following day Sebutape samples were collected from the right posterior buccal maxillary quadrant. At this point the subjects were instructed to reinstitute their normal oral hygiene practices, received a scaling/prophy and were exited from the study.

GI is a qualitative four scale based on tissue color, consistency, and bleeding on probing with scoring criteria as follows: 0 = normal gingiva; 1 = mild inflammation with no bleeding on probing; 2 = moderate inflammation with bleeding on probing, and 3 = severe inflammation with tendency for spontaneous bleeding. In this study, the entire dentition with the exception of the third molars was evaluated. For each tooth, six gingival margin areas (distobuccal, buccal, mesiobuccal, distolingual, lingual, and mesiolingual) were scored using adequate light, a mouth mirror and a periodontal probe. The probe was inserted approximately 1–2 mm into the gingival sulcus and passed from interproximal to interproximal. One aspect (either buccal or lingual) of each tooth in a quadrant was probed/skimmed and then graded before continuing to the next quadrant. Each of the six tooth surfaces was given a GI score of 0–3. A subject's full mouth score was determined by summing the scores and dividing by the number of sites examined. In addition, the number of bleeding sites is derived from the total number of sites scored as 2 and 3.

The II for gingival inflammation has been employed extensively in animal models to measure the extent of gingival inflammation with respect to the gingival margin. The extent of inflammation represented by redness, swelling, and/or broken capillaries is measured in millimeters with a periodontal probe from the free gingival margin to the junction where the visible signs of inflammation are absent. Teeth were graded by buccal or lingual surfaces (two surfaces per tooth). Measurements were made with the probe perpendicular to the free gingival margin. The point of maximum inflammation extent on each tooth surface was used to define the score for the tooth surface.

Sebutape® sampling is a novel method used to sample epithelial pro-inflammatory cytokine levels. Sebutape® is a commercially available (CuDerm) lipophilic microporous film/adhesive patch designed specifically to noninvasively sample skin surfaces for sebaceous secretions. It has been reapplied to sample surface keratinocyte cytokine levels in skin [24, 25]. This was the first application of this sampling method in the oral cavity. The Sebutape® was supplied as 20 × 28 mm patches. In this study, Sebutape® patches were bissected yielding patches that were 10 × 28 mm in size for use in the oral cavity. Sebutape® samples were collected from the attached gingiva overlying teeth 2–6 of the right maxillary posterior buccal quadrant. Prior to collecting the Sebutape® sample, the area was isolated with cotton rolls and dried with a gentle stream of air to prevent salivary contamination. The Sebutape® was applied with direct pressure to the attached gingiva including the free gingival margin and interdental papilla in the region of interest for 60 s. The sampling tape was always handled with gloves and locking forceps by the clinician to prevent cross-contamination of the sampling strip with cytokine. Care was taken to place the sampling strip so that the tape only contacted the gingival region of interest during the sampling process. Upon removal, the Sebutape® strip was stored on dry ice in a glass scintillation vial until it could be transferred to a –70 °C freezer. For the cytokine analysis, the tapes were returned to room temperature, extracted by sonicating in 1 ml of Dulbecco's phosphate-buffered saline (DPBS, Gibco BRL, Grand Island, N.Y.) for 10 min and assayed for IL-1α and IL-1β using commercially available enzyme-linked immunoabsorbant assay in accordance with the manufacturer's instructions (ELISA, R&D Systems, Minneapolis, Minn.).

These cytokine ELISA assays employ a quantitative sandwich enzyme technique. Briefly, 96-well microtiter plates are coated with a cytokine specific monoclonal antibody. Human cytokine standards (0–250 pg/ml) and Sebutape®-extracted samples were pipeted (200 µl) into the wells of the microtiter plate and incubated for 2 h at room temperature. The wells were then washed 3 times with 400 µl of DPBS to remove unbound protein. The plate wells were then incubated with 200 µl of cytokine specific polyclonal horseradish peroxidase conjugated antibody for 1 h at room temperature. The wells were again washed 3 times with 400 µl of DPBS to remove unbound antibody and exposed with a substrate solution. The color reaction was stopped with 2 *N* sulfuric acid and then the optical density of the yellow product quantitated using a spectrophotometer (450 nm minus background wavelength at 570 nm). The average reading for each standard was plotted vs. concentration and fitted by best fit linear regression analysis. The concentration of IL-1α and IL-1β from the Sebutape® extracts were calculated from the standard curves for each control cytokine.

Results

A total of 10 subjects participated in this study. There were 5 males and 5 females who were a mean (± standard error) of 36.9 ± 2.29 (range 28–46) years old. At baseline, these subjects exhibited moderate gingivitis with a mean GI of 1.10 ± 0.05 and a mean number of bleeding sites of 31.3 ± 5.1.

In general, multiple examiners using different clinical indices observed a statistically significant reduction in gingival inflammation in period 2 following

Table 1. Reduction in gingival inflammation following a scaling/prophy (mean ± SE)

Method	Period 1	Period 2	Reduction, %	p value[1]
GI score	1.10 ± 0.05	0.95 ± 0.07	13	0.003
Bleeding sites, n	31.3 ± 5.1	18.2 ± 3.5	43	< 0.001
II score	1.44 ± 0.17	0.89 ± 0.12	38	0.006

[1] Matched paired t test.

Table 2. Increase in gingival inflammation following cessation of oral hygiene for 14 days (mean ± SE)

Method	Period 2	Period 3	Increase, %	p value[1]
GI score	0.95 ± 0.07	1.25 ± 0.07	32	< 0.001
Bleeding sites, n	18.2 ± 3.5	51.2 ± 8.21	217	< 0.001
II score	0.89 ± 0.12	1.29 ± 0.07	45	0.003

[1] Matched paired t test.

a prophy as compared to period 1. For GI, the examiner observed a statistically significant 13% reduction in GI at period 2 following a scaling/prophy as compared to period 1 (table 1). Consistent with this observation, the examiner observed a statistically significant 43% reduction in the number of gingival bleeding sites from period 1 to period 2 (table 1). A second examiner utilizing the II also observed a statistically significant 38% reduction in gingival inflammation.

In contrast, multiple examiners with different indices observed a statistically significant increase in gingival inflammation in period 3 following cessation of oral hygiene as compared to period 2. For GI, the examiner observed a statistically significant increase in GI of 32% at period 3 following cessation of oral hygiene as compared to period 2 (table 2). In addition, the examiner observed a statistically significant increase in the number of gingival bleeding sites of 217% at period 3 (table 2). The second examiner utilizing the II also observed a statistically significant increase in gingival inflammation of 45%.

Sebutape® sampling of epithelial cytokines was performed during both period 2 and period 3. Consistent with the clinical results, substantial increases

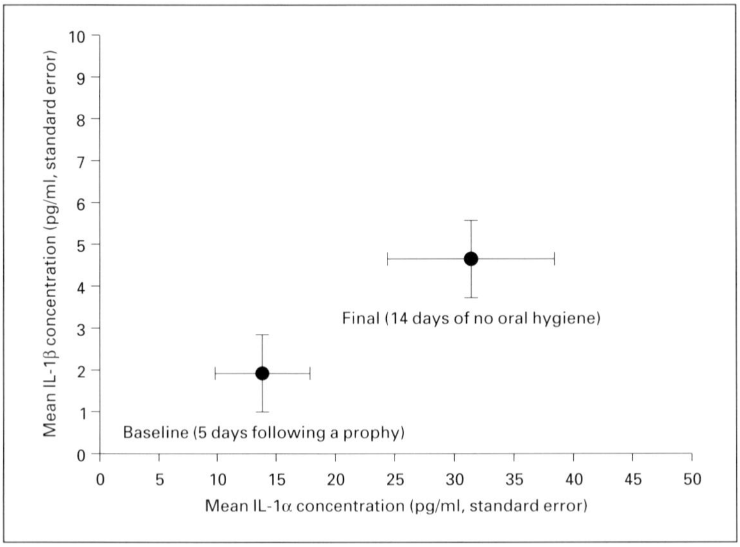

Fig. 1. Change in IL-1 concentration in 14-day experimental gingivitis.

Table 3. Increase in cytokine concentration following cessation of oral hygiene for 14 days (mean ± SE)

Method	Period 2	Period 3	Increase, %	p value[1]
IL-1α	13.81 ± 3.98	31.30 ± 6.97	127	0.001
IL-1β	1.94 ± 0.94	4.64 ± 0.92	139	0.065

[1] Matched paired t test.

in cytokine levels were observed. For IL-1α, the mean concentration of cytokine increased from 13.81 pg/ml at period 2 to 31.30 pg/ml at period 3 (table 3; fig. 1). This represented a statistically significant 127% increase in IL-1α during the cessation of oral hygiene phase of this study. For IL-1β, the mean concentration of cytokine increased from 1.94 pg/ml at period 2 to 4.64 pg/ml at period 3 (table 3; fig. 1). This represented a 139% increase in IL-1β during the cessation of oral hygiene phase of this study that was not statistically significant. Furthermore, 9 of 10 subjects had increased IL-1α and IL-1β levels from period 2 to period 3, demonstrating that the epithelial cytokine increases observed in the experimental model were a general effect that occurred across the observed

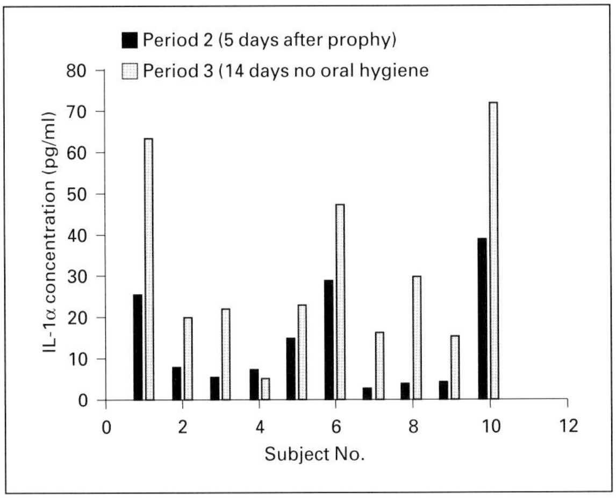

Fig. 2. Change in IL-1α concentrations by subject.

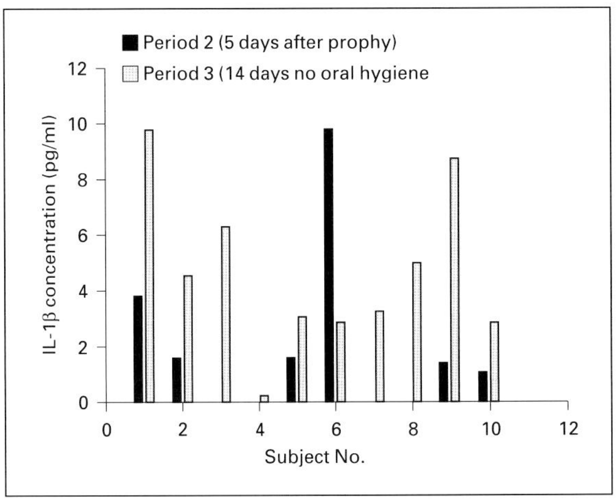

Fig. 3. Change in IL-1β concentrations by subject.

population (fig. 2, 3). Three of 10 subjects had IL-1β levels that, while present, were found to be below the limit of detection (<0.1 pg) of the IL-1β ELISA method at period 2. For the purpose of all analyses, these three data observations were conservatively treated as 0.1 pg/ml.

The clinical implications of alterations in epithelial IL-1 concentrations were further examined by correlating clinical presentation to cytokine concentration using linear regression analyses. The within-subject variability and

Table 4. Correlation of gingival cytokine levels to clinical inflammation signs

	Number of bleeding sites		Mean inflammation index	
	IL-1α	IL-1β	IL-1α	IL-1β
Gingival area sampled	r = 0.93	r = 0.90	r = 0.93	r = 0.86
Whole mouth	r = 0.93	r = 0.90	r = 0.94	r = 0.86

Linear regression analyses were performed using logarithm transformation of IL-1α and IL-1β values and were corrected for within-subject variation and period effect.

period effect were included in the regression models. The results showed that subject IL-1α and IL-1β concentrations were positively correlated to the number of clinical bleeding sites from the region of gingiva sampled with Sebutape® with r = 0.93 and 0.90, respectively (table 4, fig. 4). Linear regression analyses also demonstrated a strong positive correlation between the mean II score from the region of gingiva sampled with Sebutape® and IL-1α (r = 0.93), as well as IL-1β (r = 0.86). Consistent with these observations, IL-1α and IL-1β concentrations were positively correlated to whole mouth number of bleeding sites and mean II scores. These data suggest that cytokine levels are reasonable surrogates of the level of inflammation of not only the region of gingiva sampled, but also the gingiva of the whole mouth.

Discussion

The results of this study demonstrate that Sebutape® sampling of gingiva in the oral cavity for cytokine levels offers an alternative noninvasive sampling technique to GCF collection for monitoring cytokine changes during gingival inflammation. In this method, the Sebutape® is placed in direct contact with a defined area of attached and marginal gingiva. In theory, it collects primarily keratinocyte-derived cytokine, although there is probably some carryover cytokine from the GCF. The results of this study support this theory as the mean levels of IL-1α recovered were an order of magnitude higher than those of IL-1β. IL-1α has been shown to be the predominant form of IL-1 synthesized and stored by keratinocytes [12–14, 16]. In contrast to the Sebutape® method, sampling of GCF (a serum exudate/transudate derived from the underlying connective tissue) is likely different in that the cytokines in GCF are thought to be primarily of connective tissue orgin via macrophage, monocyte, and neutrophil secretion with IL-1β the predominant form of IL-1.

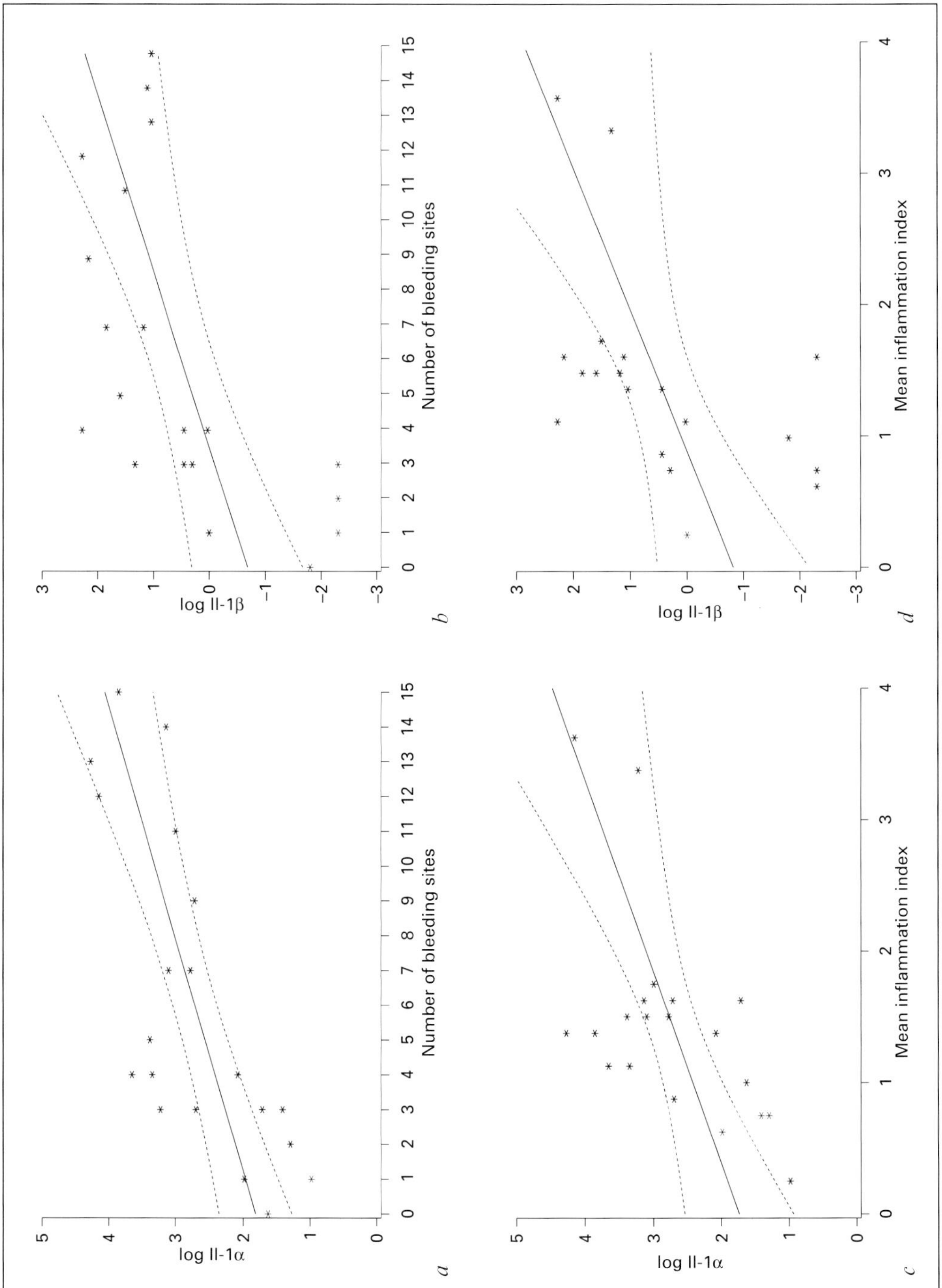
log Il-1α
Number of bleeding sites
a
log Il-1β
Number of bleeding sites
b
log Il-1α
Mean inflammation index
c
log Il-1β
Mean inflammation index
d

4

The principal role of keratinocytes is to provide a physical barrier (epithelium) between the host and environment. However, when epithelial damage or insult occurs, keratinocytes may play an active role in defense against microbial infection through the production and release of proinflammatory molecules, including IL-1. This release of IL-1 is likely the result of keratinocyte cell membrane damage, as keratinocytes do not appear to actively secrete IL-1α or IL-1β [16]. Recently, adherent streptococci have been shown to induce keratinocyte cell membrane damage in vitro and in parallel upregulate IL-1 transcription [28]. It has been hypothesized that the initial response in the inflammatory cascade during gingival inflammation is the keratinocyte release of early inflammatory mediators such as IL-1 in the gingival epithelium [21]. This 'first wave' response to microbial challenge potentially precedes and initiates the macrophage and monocyte release of cytokines and other pro-inflammatory mediators in the underlying connective tissue leading to an amplification and propagation of the inflammatory response. In fact, in cutaneous studies the release of IL-1α from basal keratinocytes in vivo is sufficient to both initiate and mediate cutaneous inflammation in vivo [29, 30]. Collectively, these data support the prominent role of keratinocyte cells in the initiation of inflammation in the oral cavity.

Mechanistically IL-1 exerts both local effects in the epithelium and distal effects in the underlying connective tissue. Keratinocyte-derived IL-1 stimulates expression of IL-6 and IL-8 within keratinocytes, which are involved in the amplification of local inflammation through the activation of lymphocytes and keratinocytes and recruitment of neutrophils [16, 28]. Both IL-1 and IL-6 have been shown to penetrate reconstructed basement membrane, supporting the ability of epithelial-derived cytokines to exert distal effects in the underlying connective tissue [31]. Other coordinated pro-inflammatory properties of IL-1 include stimulation of prostaglandin and thromboxane synthesis, stimulation of collagenase and protease production, potentiation of neutrophil degranulation and superoxide production, enhancement of endothelial cell leukocyte adhesion, and stimulation of fibroblast and keratinocyte proliferation [9–11]. In addition, IL-1 has the ability to stimulate inhibition of bone formation and enhancement of bone resorption, which in conjunction with the stimulation of collagenase and protease production may be related to destruction of the periodontium in periodontitis [4–8].

Previous studies have demonstrated that IL-1β from GCF increases during gingival inflammation prior to the onset of clinical signs of gingivitis [21, 22].

Fig. 4. Relationship of clinical inflammation to epithelial cytokine levels. *a* Area-specific bleeding sites vs. IL-1α. *b* Area-specific bleeding sites vs. IL-1β. *c* Area-specific inflammation index vs. IL-1α. *d* Area-specific inflammation index vs. IL-1β.

These studies have reported increases in cytokine level after only 3 days in an experimental gingivitis study. Pilot work in 4 subjects with Sebutape® also demonstrated that increases in both IL-1α and IL-1β can be seen after 3 days (unpublished data). In this study, increases in IL-1α and IL-1β were observed during the developmental of experimental gingivitis and paralleled increases observed in inflammation and bleeding at 7 days. In addition, positive correlations between IL-1α and clinical signs of inflammation (visual inflammation and gingival bleeding) were observed. Given the in vitro and in vivo pro-inflammatory effects of IL-1 and the positive correlations between IL-1 and clinical inflammation observed in this study as well as others, IL-1 appears to be a reasonable surrogate marker for the initiation and progression of gingival inflammation.

References

1 Alexander MB, Damoulis PD: The role of cytokines in the pathogenesis of periodontal disease. Curr Opin Periodont 1994;1:39–53.
2 Dinarello CA: Biology of interleukin 1. FASEB J 1988;2:108–115.
3 March CJ, Mosley B, Larsen A, Cerretti DP, Braedt GP, Price V, Gillis S, Henney CS, Kronheim SR, Grabstein K: Cloning, sequence and expression of two distinct human interleukin-1 complementary DNAs. Nature 1985;315:641–647.
4 Stashenko P, Dewhirst FE, Peros WJ, Kent RL, Age JM: Synergistic interactions between interleukin 1, tumor necrosis factor, and lymphotoxin in bone resorption. J Immunol 1987;138:1464–1468.
5 Stashenko P, Dewhirst FE, Rooney ML, Desjardins LA, Heeley JD: Interleukin-1β is a potent inhibitor of bone formation in vitro. J Bone Miner Res 1987;2:559–565.
6 Nguyen L, Dewhirst FE, Hauschka PV, Stashenko P: Interleukin-1β stimulates bone resorption and inhibits bone formation in vivo. Lymphokine Cytokine Res 1991;10:15–21.
7 Gowen M, Nedwin GE, Mundy GR: Preferential inhibition of cytokine stimulated bone resorption by recombinant interferon gamma. J Bone Miner Res 1986;1:469–474.
8 Tatakis DN: Interleukin-1 bone metabolism: A review. J Periodontol 1993;64:416–431.
9 Mizel SB, Dayer JM, Krane SM, Mergenhagen SE: Stimulation of rheumatoid synovial cell collagenase and prostaglandin production by partially purified lymphocyte activation factor (interleukin 1). Proc Natl Acad Sci USA 1981;78:2474–2477.
10 Bevilacqua MP, Pober JS, Wheeler ME, Cotran RS, Grimbrone MA Jr: Interleukin 1 acts on cultured human vascular endothelium to increase the adhesion of polymorphonuclear leukocytes, monocytes, and related leukocyte cell lines. J Clin Invest 1985;76:2003–2011.
11 Schmidt JA, Mizel SB, Cohen D, Green I: Interleukin 1, a potential regulator of fibroblast proliferation. J Immunol 1982;128:2177–2182.
12 Johnson GK, Poore TK, Squier CA, Wertz PW, Reinhardt RA, Vincent SD: Prostaglandin E_2 and interleukin-1 levels in smokeless tobacco-induced oral mucosal lesions. J Periodont Res 1994;29:430–438.
13 Johnson GK, Poore TK, Payne JB, Organ CC: Effect of smokeless tobacco extract on human gingival keratinocyte levels of prostaglandin E_2 and interleukin-1. J Periodontol 1996;67:116–124.
14 Johnson GK, Organ CC: Prostaglandin E_2 and interleukin-1 concentrations in nicotine-exposed oral keratinocytes cultures. J Periodont Res 1997;32:447–454.
15 Cassatella M: The production of cytokines by polymorphonuclear neutrophils. Immunol Today 1995;16:21–26.

16 Kupper TS: The activated keratinocyte: A model for inducible cytokine production by non-bone marrow-derived cells in cutaneous inflammatory and immune responses. J Invest Dermatol 1990; 94(suppl 6):146–150.
17 Hauser C, Saurat JH, Schmitt A, Jaunin F, Dayer JM: Interleukin-1α is present in normal human epidermis. J Immunol 1986;136:3317–3323.
18 Brecx MC, Schlegel K, Gehr P, Lang NP: Comparison between histological and clinical parameters during human experimental gingivitis. J Periodont Res 1987;22:50–57.
19 Brecx MC, Lehmann B, Siegwart CM, Gehr P, Lang NP: Observations on the initial stages of healing following human experimental gingivitis. A clinical and morphometric study. J Clin Periodontol 1988; 15:123–129.
20 Kinane DF, Winstanley FP, Adonogianaki E, Moughal NA: Bioassay of interleukin 1 (IL-1) in human gingival crevicular fluid during experimental gingivitis. Arch Oral Biol 1992;37:153–156.
21 Heasman PA, Collins JG, Offenbacher S: Changes in crevicular fluid levels in interleukin 1β, leukotriene B_4, prostaglandin E_2, thromboxane B_2 and tumor necrosis factor α in experimental gingivitis in humans. J Periodont Res 1993;28:241–247.
22 Jotwani R, Avila R, Kim BO, Iacopino AM, Cutler CW: The effects of an antiseptic mouthrinse on subclinical gingivitis in IL-1 genotype-positive and -negative humans (abstract 2320). J Dent Res 1998;77:921.
23 Lamster IB, Grbic JT: Diagnosis of periodontal disease based on analysis of the host response. Periodont 2000 1995;7:83–99.
24 Pagnoni A, Kligman AM, Gammal SE, Stoudemayer T: Determination of density of follicles on various regions of the face by cyanoacrylate biopsy: Correlation with sebum output. Br J Dermatol 1994;131:862–865.
25 Imayama S, Shimozono Y, Urabe A, Hori Y: A simple method for measuring the amount of Immunoglobulin A secreted onto the skin surface. Acta Derm Venereol 1995;75:212–217.
26 Silness J, Loe H: Periodontal disease in pregnancy. II. Correlation between oral hygiene and periodontal condition. Acta Odontol Scand 1964;22:121–127.
27 Donovan-Brand R, Snider AG, Brown KK, Pratt JL, Hausmann E, Buchanan W: Endotoxin changes during natural periodontitis progression in dogs (abstract 775). J Dent Res 1997;76:110.
28 Kondo S, Kooshesh, Sauder D: Penetration of keratinocyte-derived cytokines into basement membrane. J Cell Physiol 1997;171:190–195.
29 Wang B, Ruiz N, Pentland A, Caparon M: Keratinocyte proinflammatory responses to adherent and nonadherent group A streptococci. Infect Immun 1997;65:2119–2126.
30 Groves RW, Mizutani H, Kieffer JD, Kupper TS: Inflammatory skin disease in transgenic mice that express high levels of interleukin 1 alpha in basal epidermis. Proc Natl Acad Sci USA 1995; 92:11874–11878.
31 Groves RW, Rauschmayr T, Nakamura K, Sarkar S, Williams IR, Kupper TS: Inflammatory and hyperproliferative skin disease in mice that express elevated levels of the IL-1 receptor (type I) on epidermal keratinocytes. Evidence that IL-1-inducible secondary cytokines produced by keratinocytes in vivo can cause skin disease. J Clin Invest 1996;98:336–344.

Dr. Aaron R. Biesbrock, Procter & Gamble Company,
8700 Mason-Montgomery Road, Mason, OH 45040–9462 (USA)
Tel. +1 513 622-0316, Fax +1 513 622-1560, E-Mail biesbrock.ar@pg.com

Faller RV (ed): Assessment of Oral Health.
Monogr Oral Sci. Basel, Karger, 2000, vol 17, pp 32–55

Imaging of the Oral Cavity Using Optical Coherence Tomography

Bill W. Colston, Jr.[a], *Matthew J. Everett*[a], *Ujwal S. Sathyam*[a], *Luiz B. DaSilva*[a], *Linda L. Otis*[b]

[a] Lawrence Livermore National Laboratory, Livermore, Calif., and
[b] University of Connecticut Health Center, Stanford, Conn. USA

Abstract

Optical coherence tomography is a new method for noninvasively imaging internal tooth and soft tissue microstructure. The intensity of backscattered light is measured as a function of depth in the tissue. Low coherence interferometry is used to selectively remove the component of backscattered signal that has undergone multiple scattering events, resulting in very high resolution images (<15μm). Lateral scanning of the probe beam across the biological tissue is then used to generate a 2-D intensity plot, similar to ultrasound images. This imaging method provides information that is currently unobtainable by any other means, making possible such diverse applications as diagnosis of periodontal disease, caries detection, and evaluation of restoration integrity. This chapter presents an overview of this exciting new imaging technique and its current application to dental diagnosis.

Introduction

Optical coherence tomography (OCT) is a new method for noninvasively imaging internal tooth and soft tissue microstructure. This imaging method provides information that is currently unobtainable by any other means, making possible such diverse applications as diagnosis of periodontal diseases, caries detection, and evaluation of restoration integrity. This chapter presents an overview of this exciting new imaging technique and its current application to dental diagnosis.

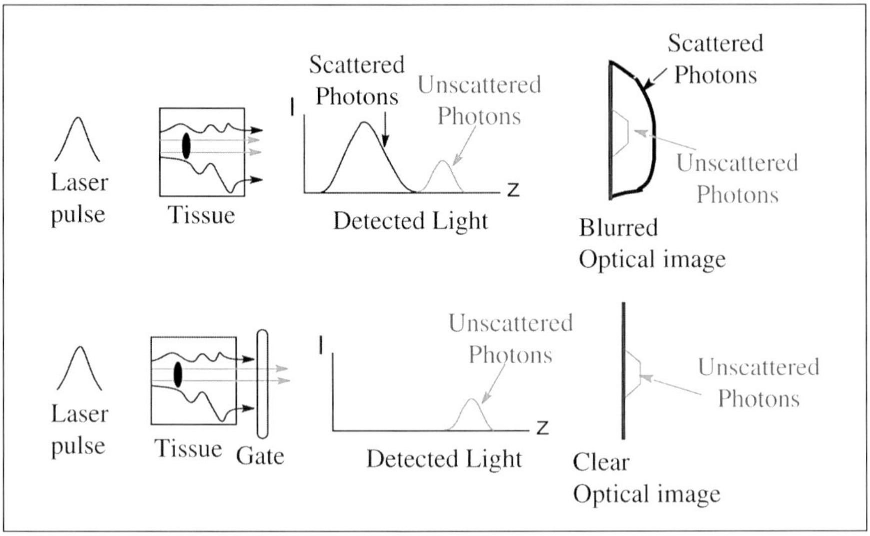

Fig. 1. Optical imaging through a highly turbid media such as biological tissue often results in blurred images due to scattering events in the media. Removal of the light that becomes highly scattered allows high resolution imaging to occur.

Optical Imaging of Biological Tissue

The characteristic interaction of light photons with biological tissue can be used to create diagnostic images. The highest quality image information is contained in the portion of the detected light that is relatively unscattered and therefore travels the most direct path through the tissue. Unfortunately, scattering events predominate when light interacts with biological tissue. Thus, without scatter-reduction techniques, signal-to-noise ratios (unscattered to scattered components) limit axial resolution in optical imaging methods to no better than 1 cm. Scatter-reduction methods, however, such as time-resolved systems (fig. 1), can achieve millimeter resolutions by gating the unscattered (early arriving) from the scattered (delayed) photons. Other scatter-reduction methodologies that have been explored include cross-correlation techniques [1], time-delayed coincidence counting [2], Kerr gating [3], holographic gating [4], Raman gating [5], and streak cameras [6]. These methodologies, however, have not been optimized to provide sub-millimeter resolution of structures in biological tissue, and are less easily adapted to a clinical environment.

OCT and its one-dimensional analog, optical coherence domain reflectometry (OCDR), rely on low coherence interferometry to selectively remove the scattered component of the reflected light. OCT can be performed using broadband light sources and fiber optics, obviating the need for more complicated ultrashort pulsed laser systems. OCT instruments can thus be developed that are clinically practical and capable of producing in vivo cross-sectional images of tissue microstructure with sub-millimeter resolution.

History of OCT

OCDR was first developed as a high resolution ranging technique for characterization of optical components [7]. A group at MIT headed by Dr. James Fujimoto combined transverse scanning with a fiber optic OCDR system to produce the first OCT cross-sectional images of biological microstructure [8]. The first clinical application of OCT was ophthalmic imaging to establish the diagnosis of retinal macular diseases [9]. Although OCT has high resolution, the imaging depth is relatively limited (1–3 mm) in the majority of biological tissues. Extraocular studies have focused on regions where optical access is unrestricted such as the skin [10], or can be reached by catheters or endoscopic probes [11]. These imaging depths are also sufficient for visualizing clinically relevant internal tissue microstructures in the oral cavity. Our group has pioneered the use of OCT in dentistry and demonstrated its usefulness for a variety of applications [12, 13]. Recently, this initial research has been complemented by other groups performing OCT imaging studies of dental tissues [14, 15].

Dental Applications of OCT

Currently, dentists evaluate the oral health of a patient through three main avenues: visual/tactile examination; periodontal probing, and radiographic imaging. The mainstay of periodontal diagnosis is conventional probing. Unfortunately, as a diagnostic technique periodontal probing is moderately imprecise. Errors associated with current probing methods decrease the sensitivity of clinical periodontal diagnosis and complicate research. Measurement error limits the ability to evaluate subtle differences in clinical values that may be important in early disease detection and intervention. Probing errors result from variations in insertion force, the inflammatory status of the tissue, the diameter of probe tips, and anatomical tooth contours [16, 17]. Radiographs can be used as a supplementary tool in periodontal disease diagnosis to reveal the morphological characteristics of alveolar bone. While radiographs are highly sensitive to detecting regions of alveolar bone loss, they are incapable of identifying active disease. Periodontal disease is therefore not identified until significant bone loss has occurred. Conventional radiographs, moreover, provide little information on soft tissue states. Because OCT records soft tissue contour and microstructure, it offers the potential to quantify the soft tissue changes that occur in gingivitis and periodontal diseases.

Dental caries is currently diagnosed using radiography in conjunction with visual and tactile exploration. The traditional method of caries detection, probing the teeth with a sharp dental explorer, has fallen into disfavor because it causes damage to the tooth by penetrating the enamel and may also cause microbiological cross-contamination between teeth. Although radiography uses ionizing radiation that carries the potential for detrimental biological effects, it remains an essential component of caries diagnosis. Radiography has high predictive value for detecting interproximal lesions involving the dentin. Radiography also shows a high sensitivity for detecting occlusal caries that involves dentin, although the false-positive fraction is high. The predictive value of radiography for class V or for lesions confined to the enamel is poor [18, 19]. OCT holds promise to supplement radiographic diagnosis for detecting early occlusal lesions and for quantifying enamel demineralization and class-V lesions. OCT may also prove to be more sensitive for detecting recurrent caries because the margins of restorations are imaged in tomographic sections with a higher resolution than can be obtained using current radiographic methods.

OCT therefore offers a safe, novel method to image dental microstructure for evaluation of dental health. Potential dental applications of OCT include, among others, diagnosis of periodontal diseases, detection of caries, and evaluation of dental restoration integrity. Any region of the oral cavity that is accessible and contains useful information within the first 2–3 mm of tissue can potentially benefit from this technique.

Principles of OCT Imaging

General Principles

The Michelson interferometer, first introduced by Albert Michelson in the late 18th century, is the basis for OCDR. OCDR maps the intensity of light backscattered from internal structural interfaces as a function of their axial (depth) positions. The addition of lateral scanning to a system creates a tomographic, or OCT image. A diagram of a basic fiber optic Michelson interferometer is shown in figure 2. Optical radiation from a source is split equally down the sample and reference arms of the interferometer by the fiber coupler. Backscattered light from dental tissue is then recombined with the reflection from the reference mirror and propagated to the detector from the fiber coupler. An interferometric signal is detected when the distance to the reference and sample arm reflections is matched to within the source coherence length. Axial or depth profiling of structural interfaces in the tissue is accomplished by varying the pathlength of the reference arm mirror using a scanning mirror or piezotransducer. The signal at the detector is then sent through a lock-in amplifier or bandpass filter to demodulate the interference signal. The

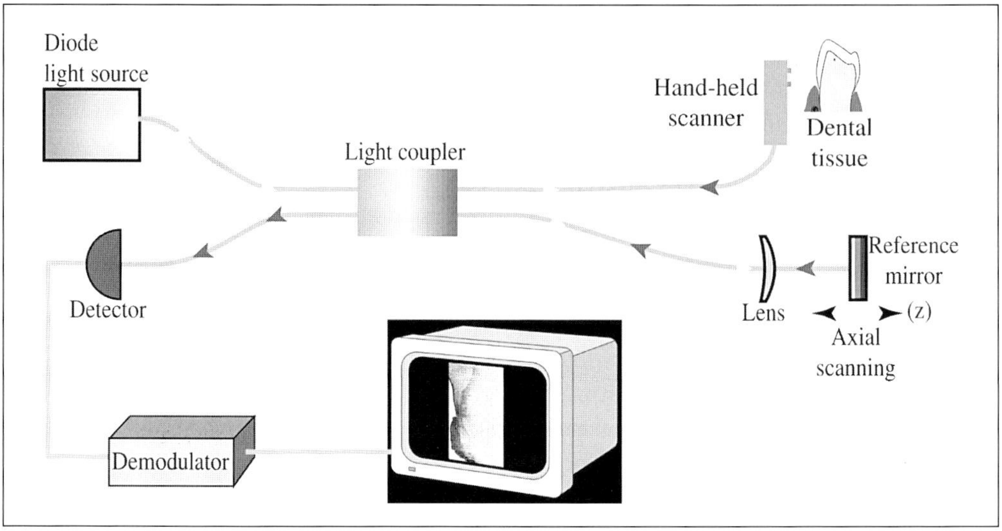

Fig. 2. Fiber optic white light Michelson interferometer.

magnitude of the demodulated interference pattern is plotted against the axial position of the reference mirror to produce a one-dimensional scan. The terminology for this depth profiling, A-Scan, has been borrowed from ultrasound technology.

Axial Resolution

The mathematical treatment of interference, coherence, and beam propagation has been developed in a number of textbooks. The subject of coherence theory is covered in great detail in the text written by Mandel and Wolf [20]. An excellent overview of basic interferometry is provided in the classic text of Born and Wolf [21], while the specific application of fiber optics and optical heterodyne detection can be found in the reference by Haus [22]. As the mathematics surrounding coherence theory is relatively complex, we refer the reader to the suggested references and only provide an intuitive understanding of the process here.

The axial resolution of an OCT system is directly related to the coherence length of the light source. The shorter the coherence length, the smaller the path length mismatch must be for an interferometric signal to be generated. Thus decreasing the source coherence length results in a higher axial (depth) resolution. Coherence length is dependent on the spectral bandwidth of the light source. Periodic distributions formed by light of different frequency

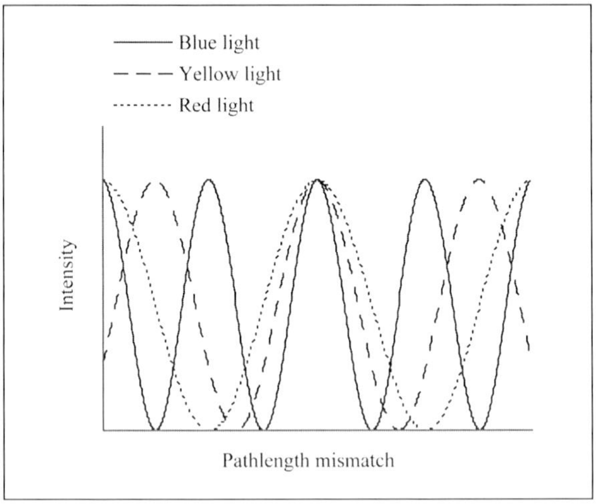

Fig. 3. Different periodicities associated with a given wavelength of light become more out of step with one another as the pathlength mismatch between the two interferometer arms increases.

components have different spatial periodicities. These periodicities become out of step as the pathlength mismatch between the interfering optical waves increases (fig. 3). Eventually, the periodic intensity distributions become so out of step that no fringe pattern is formed. The more frequency components that are present (i.e. the larger the spectral bandwidth of the source), the closer the pathlengths of the two interferometric arms must be matched for an interference pattern to occur. The axial resolution of the system is thus inversely proportional to the spectral bandwidth of the source. Low coherence sources with a broad frequency distribution are necessary if images with submillimeter resolution are to be created, since the spectral bandwidth of the source determines the accuracy of the interferometric ranging measurement. For example, a white light source (wide spectral bandwidth) would have a much higher axial resolutions than a laser (narrow bandwidth). The light sources used in dental OCT studies have relatively broad spectral bandwidths in the order of 30–60 nm, with corresponding free space axial resolutions between 10 and 20 μm.

System Sensitivity and Dynamic Range

The sensitivity of an OCT system is defined as the ratio of the light focused on the biological tissue (P_{tot}) to the minimum (P_{min}) detectable light returning from the tissue. Sensitivity is generally defined in terms of a logarithmic value (dB) as:

$$\text{Sensitivity (dB)} = 10 \cdot \log\left(\frac{P_{tot}}{P_{min}}\right).$$

The ability to recombine the weak reflection from the sample tissue with the strong reflection from the reference arm mirror results in excellent system sensitivity. This sensitivity is typically 90–110 dB. This translates to minimum detectable reflections in the order of 10^{-9} to 10^{-11} of the incident power. If the power on the sample was 70 μW, for example, an OCT system with a sensitivity of 90 dB could detect 70 fW of reflected light. This high level of sensitivity is achieved through the use of electronic filters that extract the desired signal from the noise.

The dynamic range of an OCT system is defined as the level of light returning from the tissue that causes the detector system to saturate over the minimum detectable power. The highest achievable dynamic range occurs when the overall noise of the system is limited by the shot noise. Shot noise is simply the standard deviation of random intensity fluctuations of light and charge at the photodetector, and scales with the square root of the photocurrent power. The backscattered light from the sample is assumed to be negligibly small compared to the reference reflection power, since the intensity of backscattered light from a highly scattering media such as biological tissue is very low. The dynamic range is defined logarithmically and is 40–60 dB in a typical OCT system.

Imaging Depth

Imaging depth, as mentioned in the Introduction, is a critical characteristic of OCT imaging. An understanding of this basic limitation is necessary before the clinical usefulness of OCT systems can be evaluated. One convenient and relatively simple model for determining the factors that govern OCT imaging depth is the radiative transport theory. This analytical approach describes light propagation through a biological medium and is based solely on the intensity and spectral features of the propagated optical radiation. The radiative transport theory ignores effects associated with the wave nature of light (such as interference, dispersion, etc.). Absorption and scattering characteristics of a given tissue are represented by the absorption coefficient (μ_a) and scattering coefficient (μ_s) in units of inverse optical pathlength. These parameters can be intuitively understood by realizing that they are inversely proportional to the absorption and scattering mean free paths, where the mean free path is defined as the average distance a photon travels in the tissue before undergoing an absorption or scattering event.

The intensity of coherent backscattered light from a highly scattering media such as biological tissue decays exponentially as a function of depth

[23]. The attenuation of the backscattered light, measurable as incident versus reflected power at the sample arm (P_{out}/P_{in}), can be expressed as a function of optical penetration depth (L), such that:

$$\frac{P_{out}}{P_{in}} = \exp[-2(\mu_a + \mu_s)L].$$

This equation is simply a modified version of the familiar Beer-Lambert Law used in optical transmission spectroscopy, which states that absorption of a given analyte in a dilute medium is logarithmically related to the concentration of that analyte as a function of optical penetration depth. In the case of OCT, however, particles that scatter light can be treated as absorbers, since the coherence gating and confocal nature of the OCT system theoretically eliminate the multiply-scattered photons.

Improvements in source power have a limited effect on the imaging depth of an OCT system since this term is outside the exponential term of the signal to noise calculation. This places a quantum limit on the maximum imaging depth achievable with an OCT system, assuming that the optical power of the system is limited by the damage threshold of the tissue [24]. Efforts to improve this imaging depth OCT system must focus on reducing the absorption and scattering coefficients of the biological tissue by selection of an appropriate source wavelength.

The major absorbers in soft tissue are hemoglobin, melanin, and water. The spectral region from approximately 600 to 1,400 nm is often called the 'window of opportunity' in medical photonics, since optical absorption is minimized in this band and scattering becomes the dominant loss mechanism. The scattering properties of tissue are much more difficult to quantify than the absorption properties. Particle size, geometry, and relative index of refraction differences must all be considered [25]. The general wavelength dependence of the scattering coefficient has, however, been determined for a variety of biological tissues [26, 27] and can be expressed as:

$$\mu_s \propto \frac{1}{\lambda_0^n},$$

where n varies from 2 to 4 and λ_0 is the central wavelength of the optical source. Thus, in a system dominated by scattering alone, longer wavelengths have much greater penetration depths than shorter wavelengths.

The scattering and absorption properties of selected tissues in the oral cavity have been determined [28]. These investigators found that the absorption coefficients of enamel and dentin were negligible compared to their scattering coefficients. The scattering coefficient for enamel was significantly reduced at higher wavelengths ($n = 3$) while there was no significant wavelength depend-

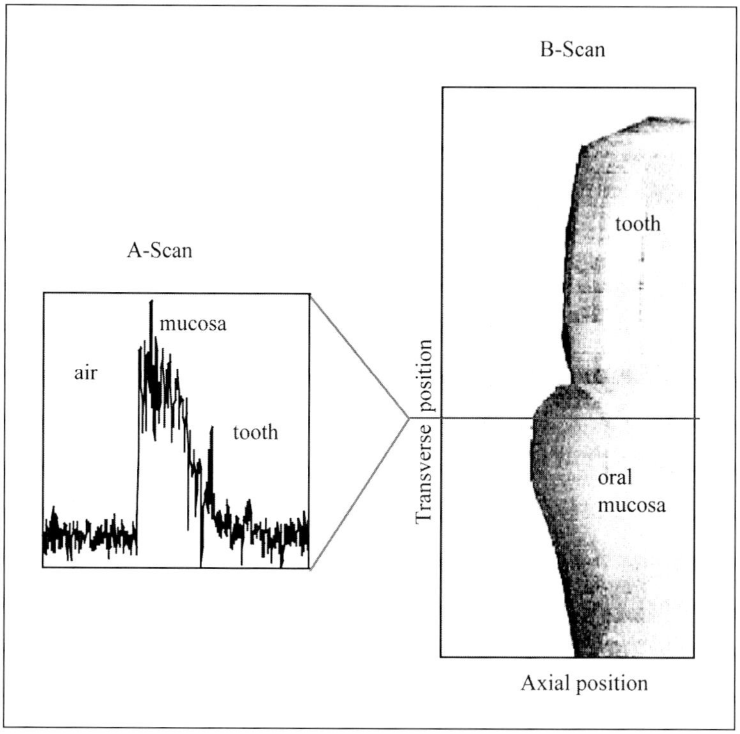

Fig. 4. Two-dimensional A-scans (axial position vs. reflectance) are stacked sequentially to create a cross-sectional intensity plot, or B-scan image.

ence (n = 0) for dentin. Although no soft tissue measurements were made, comparisons with similar tissue types (connective tissue) typically yields values between n = 3 and n = 4 with negligible absorption at wavelengths between 850 and 1,400 nm. The optical wavelength of choice for current dental OCT systems is 1,310 nm.

Transverse Scanning and Intraoral Handpieces

In OCT, a cross-sectional image is produced by transversely scanning the beam across the tissue and collecting a reflectance versus depth profile at each transverse location. The reflectance intensities are then recorded digitally on a grayscale image as a function of their transverse and axial locations (fig. 4).

The lateral resolution of an OCT system is limited by the size of the focused beam on the tissue and determined by the spacing between individual axial scans (A-scans). The spacing between scans is given by the ratio of the speed with which the sample arm collection optics are laterally scanned across

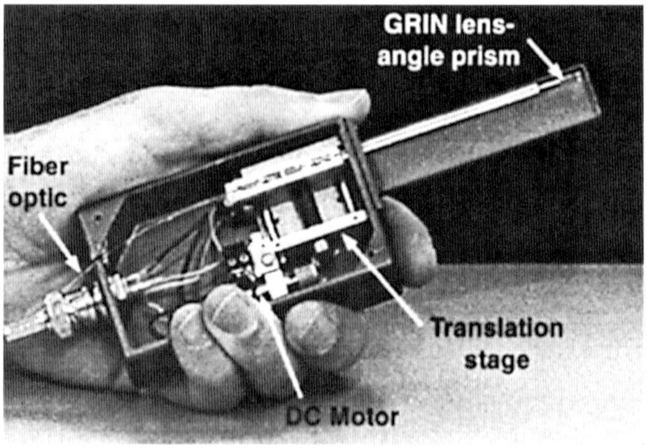

Fig. 5. Intraoral OCT handpiece (one dimension of lateral scanning).

the tissue over the rate at which A-scans are collected. The lateral resolution is typically between 20 and 100 μm. The minimum waist size of the beam at the focus (w_0) can be measured or determined by Gaussian optical theory. The depth over which the beam remains relatively focused is defined as twice the Rayleigh range ($z_{Rayleigh}$). Increasing the Rayleigh range means sacrificing transverse resolution, since $z_{Rayleigh} \propto w_0^2$. Optimum OCT systems are designed to minimize the depth of focus by setting the Rayleigh range to half the value of the measured penetration depth.

A variety of different intraoral optical prototype handpieces have been designed to access the oral cavity. The two primary design considerations include comfortable access to the human oral cavity and a method for transversely scanning the sample arm to perform cross-sectional imaging. Comfortable access can be achieved by miniaturizing the sample arm collection optics. One example of an intraoral handpiece design is shown in figure 5. The collection optics include a gradient refractive index (GRIN) lens/angle prism combination mounted on the end of the sample arm single mode fiber optic. Light emerging from the fiber is focused by the GRIN lens to a 20-μm spot on the tissue and reflected 90° by an internal reflection from a prism. The fiber optic/GRIN lens assembly is linearly scanned parallel to the facial surface of the dental tissue. This 'side-firing' handpiece allows easy access to the posterior portion of the oral cavity.

The intraoral handpiece shown above is capable of two-dimensional (cross-sectional or B-scan) imaging. Other designs exist for performing three-dimensional scanning, where the distance between adjacent B-scans is precisely controlled [15]. This type of scanning is particularly useful where volumetric estimates of tissue density (such as location of small carious lesions) is desirable.

The limitation of these 3-D intraoral handpieces is their size: the end of the handpiece must necessarily be large enough to accommodate the maximum distance of travel for both transverse scanning directions.

Image Acquisition Time

An OCT system must have relatively rapid acquisition times to prevent motion artifacts. This is particularly relevant in a clinical setting. Motion error can lead to a loss of spatial resolution in both the axial and transverse directions. Axial movement of the patient relative to the OCT sample collection optics can result in erroneous changes in signal intensity. Since the B-scan intensity image is formed from a series of longitudinal A-scans, axial motion can also lead to misalignment of subsequent transverse scans with a resulting loss of the surface contour profile. Transverse motion error that is large relative to the image acquisition time leads to inaccuracies in the transverse resolution and nonlinear longitudinal information.

One method of minimizing these motion artifacts is to design the intraoral handpiece to be in direct contact with the sample tissue. Motion artifacts that occur under these conditions are infrequent. Those that do occur (fig. 6), however, are primarily caused by low frequency modulations between adjacent longitudinal scans due to patient or operator movement.

Standard OCT dental imaging systems take between 30 and 60 s to acquire a single B-scan image, given a 1-cm scan range with <30-μm transverse resolutions. Improvements in image acquisition time can only be accomplished by sacrificing lateral resolution, increasing the optical power of the light source, or reducing the imaging depth of the system. More extensive evaluations will need to be made in the future to determine the optimum set of parameters for a given application.

Image Artifacts Caused by Multiple Optical Paths

Strong reflections such as plastic infection control sleeves or the front interface of a tooth can cause optical echoes to appear in the OCT images. These echoes are proportional to the magnitude of their respective primary reflection peaks and are directly correlated with the source output power. Backscatter from internal tissue microstructure rarely has reflected amplitudes of >30 dB above the noise floor, so these 'coherent spikes' are only detectable at specular reflection points such as the first air/tissue interface. These echoes are created by multiple path reflections within the optical components of the OCT system. The output facets from the diode optical source, for example, can often cause these image artifacts (fig. 7). Careful selection of infection control devices and orientation of the optical intraoral handpiece with respect to the tissue being imaged can eliminate many of these artifacts.

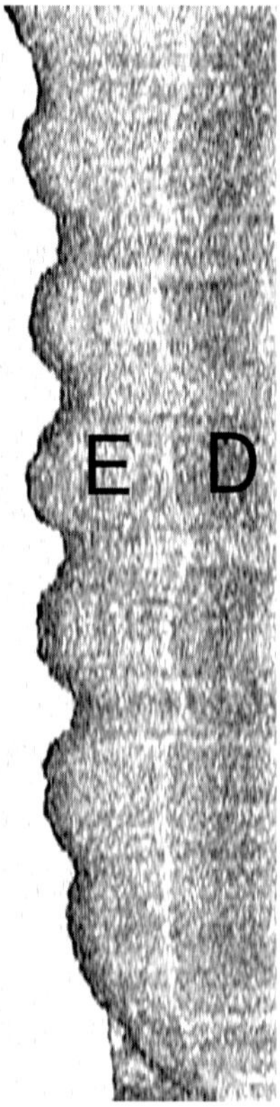

Fig. 6. Tooth surface showing motion artifacts.

Imaging in the Oral Cavity

Periodontal Tissues – In vitro Imaging

The first OCT imaging of dental structures were conducted using an animal model [12]. Selected regions from the oral cavity of 2 young pigs were imaged shortly after sacrifice using a bench-top dental OCT system. The source used in this experiment was relatively low-powered (~ 70 μW) with a net system signal-to-noise ratio of 90 dB. The axial and lateral resolution of the system was 17 and 20 μm, respectively. Histological confirmation of the OCT images was made by freezing the specimens and then slicing them axially using a diamond-tipped rotating disk. The internal tooth and soft tissue microstructure was thus exposed and the critical tooth/gingiva interface maintained. A digital camera mounted on a microscope was used to obtain photomicrographs of the sectioned teeth.

This in vitro approach had the benefit of allowing direct comparisons of the acquired OCT cross-sectional images to histology (fig. 8). The axial scale

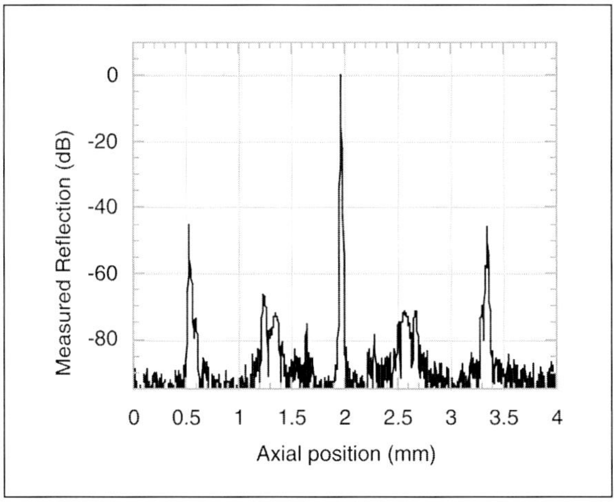

Fig. 7. A-scan of a mirror in the sample arm (central peak). Reflection peaks on the wings are artifacts created by multiple optical paths.

for the OCT image is in terms of optical pathlength and needs to be divided by the refractive index of the relevant tissue to obtain true physical dimensions, resulting in an axial compression of the image. The refractive indices for gingiva, enamel, and dentin are ~1.3, ~1.6, and ~1.5, respectively. The sulcus (S), an important reference point for determining attachment level in evaluation of periodontal diseases, is clearly visible in these early in vitro OCT images. In addition, the dento-enamel junction (DEJ), whose integrity is important in caries diagnosis, is also discernable. Although the periodontal tissues of the porcine specimens used in the study were healthy, the images demonstrated the ability of OCT to locate the tooth surface and contour beneath the gingival tissue. This was an important step in establishing the validity of this technique for dental medicine.

Periodontal Tissues – in vivo Studies

Compact dental OCT systems for clinical use now exist. These in vivo imaging systems incorporate intraoral handpiece designs that allow access to most parts of the oral cavity. An example demonstrating the type of tissue structural detail that can be obtained with these in vivo OCT systems is shown in figure 9. This image of healthy periodontal tissue was collected from the facial side of a volunteer's mandibular first premolar, and represents a 20-μm-thick cross-section of the tooth at the cervical region. No post-processing has been used in creating this image. The surface contour of this particular tissue is well represented, although slight motion artifact can be seen as modulations

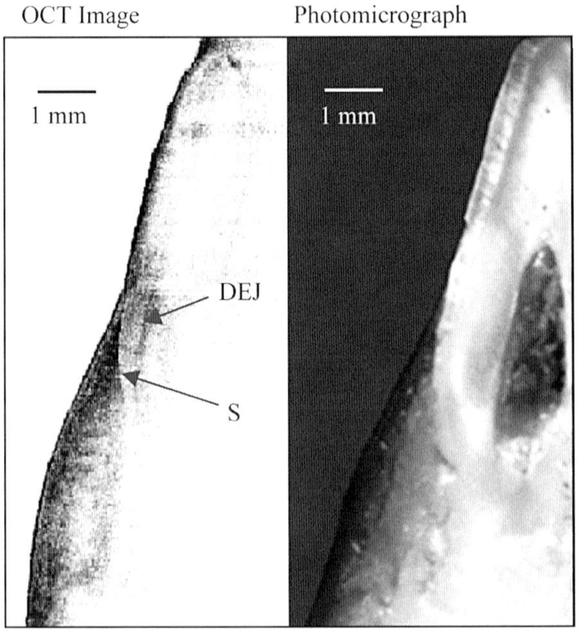

Fig. 8. Comparison of OCT and histology images for an in vitro pig's jaw showing the sulcus (S) and dentin-enamel junction (DEJ).

of the facial surface. The enamel (E) is visualized in its entirety while only approximately 1 mm of dentin is clearly visible in the image. The large mismatch in reflectivity between dentin and enamel microstructures creates a highly visible interface at the DEJ. The alveolar bone (AB) is presumptively identified as the checkered region underlying the dark epithelial layer at the base of the image. Because progression of periodontal disease results in alterations of the connective tissue architecture, the identification of these anatomical features using dental OCT is promising. More expansive clinical studies correlating OCT image characteristics with standard assessments of oral health, however, must be performed before this technique will be useful for the diagnosis of gingivitis or periodontal diseases.

Tooth Structures

The imaging depth of OCT systems in dental hard structures is superior to that in soft tissue, particularly in enamel where imaging depths of <4 mm have been successfully recorded. The OCT image (fig. 10), for example, shows a cross-section acquired in a mesial-distal direction at the level of the interprox-

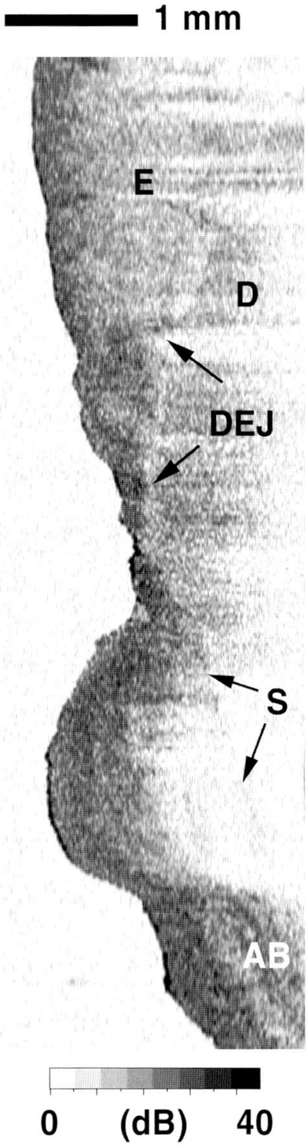

9

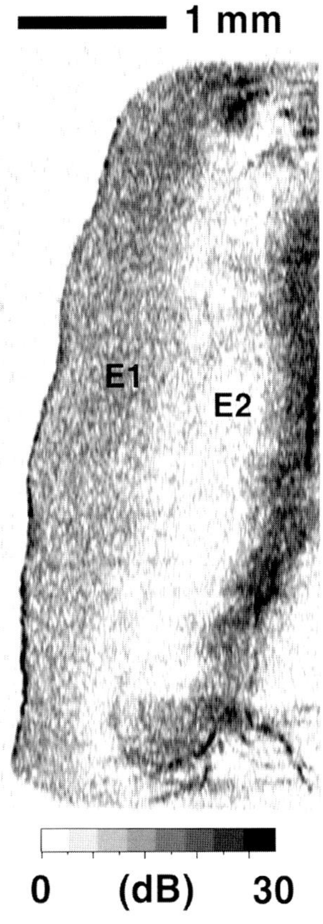

10

Fig. 9. In vitro B-scan image of a human healthy mandibular premolar taken perpendicular to the gingival margin.

Fig. 10. In vivo B-scan image of a human incisor taken parallel to the gingival margin.

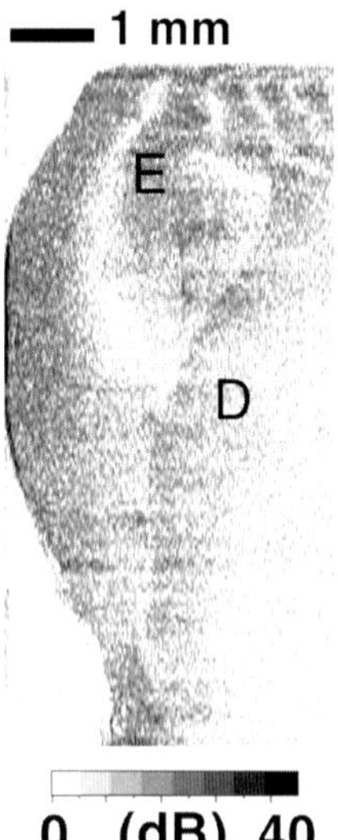

Fig. 11. In vivo B-scan image of a human tooth showing birefringence artifacts in the enamel layer (alternate black and white bands).

imal contact. Microstructural detail in the enamel layer is visible in this image, possibly correlating to prenatal (E1) and postnatal (E2) enamel formation. Enamel lamallae are also visible in this image.

Another interesting and useful facet of dental OCT imaging is the presence of birefringence effects, visible as alternating dark and light bands in the enamel layer (fig. 11). Since OCT is an interferometric technique, signal intensity is a function of the relative polarization states of the sample and reference arm reflections. Tissue that is birefringent such as enamel has an anisotropic refractive index gradient and modifies the polarization state of light passing through it. Conventional OCT systems do not have the ability to compensate for this change, resulting in image artifacts that correspond to the amount of mismatch between the polarization state of the sample and reference arm reflections. These artifacts appear primarily in contoured posterior teeth and are dependent on the relative orientation between the incident probe light and the tooth structure. The enamel prisms, made up of hydroxyapatite crystals, run like the spokes of a wheel from the DEJ to the outer enamel surface. Neighboring prisms are separated by 0.1- to 0.2-μm-wide glycoprotein prism sheaths. Enamel is birefringent because the index of refraction for light polarized along the axis of the prisms is different from the index of refraction for light polarized perpendicular to the axis. When the enamel surface is perpendicular to the incident light from the optical handpiece, the two axes of polarization of the incident light are both perpendicular to the axes of the prisms and minimal birefringence effects occur. As the contour of the tooth

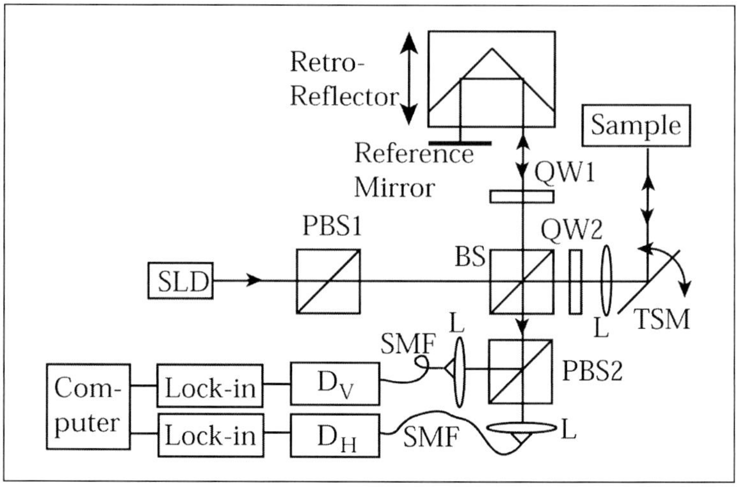

Fig. 12. Diagram of polarization-sensitive OCT (PS-OCT) system. SLD = Superluminescent diode; PBS = polarizing beam splitter; QW = quarter wave plate; BS = beamsplitter; L = lens; TSM = transverse scanning mirror; D = detector.

changes, however, the prisms become more perpendicular to the probe light and birefringence-induced artifacts appear in the OCT images.

Imaging studies have been initiated to determine if birefringence differences between normal and demineralized enamel could be used in conjunction with polarization-sensitive OCT (PS-OCT) for caries detection [29]. A representative PS-OCT system is shown in figure 12. A collimated beam from a low coherent light source is passed through a polarizer (PBS), providing horizontally polarized light. This light is then split into the reference and sample arms of the Michelson interferometer by a non-polarizing beamsplitter. A quarter wave plate set at 22.5° to horizontal in the reference arm rotates the polarization of the light by 45° upon reflection. A quarter wave plate set at 45° to horizontal in the sample arm causes circularly polarized light to be incident upon the tooth. After being reflected from the reference mirror and to tooth, the beams are recombined by the beamsplitter. A polarizing cube splits the recombined beam into its horizontal and vertical polarization components which are then coupled by single mode fiber optics into two detectors. The light from the reference arm is split evenly between the two detectors. The two polarizations of light returning from the sample arm (horizontal and vertical polarizations) are combined with the reference light at the two detectors. This provides a depth-resolved measurement of both backscattered light intensity and polarization state.

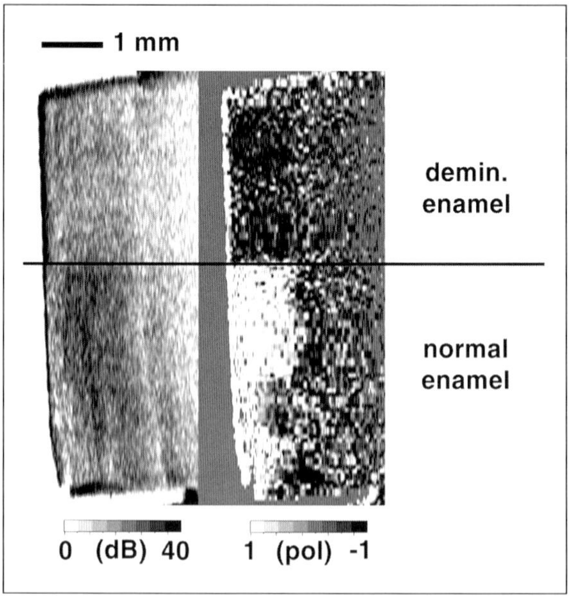

Fig. 13. Bovine block with top half of enamel demineralized. Contrast between the demineralized and normal regions is much better in the OCT phase plot (right) than in the OCT intensity plot (left).

Other investigators have attempted to measure changes in teeth birefringence using PS-OCT as a caries diagnostic [14]. Their system, however, had limited sensitivity and penetration depth, making it difficult to discriminate between birefringence and depolarization of light and resulting in inconclusive results. We have recently demonstrated, in agreement with Fried et al. [28] of UCSF, that demineralization causes depolarization of light rather than changes in birefringence. We first confirmed this ability of PS-OCT to detect caries lesions using tissue phantoms consisting of bovine enamel blocks containing artificially generated caries (fig. 13). A surface zone of demineralization approximately 50 μm thick was produced on the polished surface of half a 5×5-mm bovine enamel block, while half of the block was covered with acid-resistance varnish. The backscattering intensity (fig. 13, left) was only slightly affected by the demineralization, while the polarization state of the scattered light (fig. 13, right) clearly delineates the normal and carious enamel. The phase image is the degree of polarization of the light, defined as:

$$P = \frac{L(d) - R(d)}{L(d) + R(d)}.$$

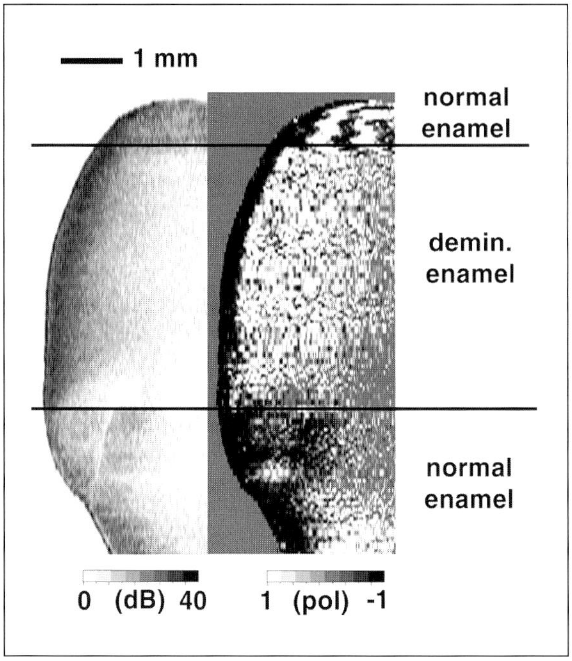

Fig. 14. Extracted tooth with a large demineralized section in the center of the enamel layer. Contrast between the demineralized and normal regions is much better in the OCT phase plot (right) than in the OCT intensity plot (left).

Here L(d) and R(d) are the amount of light returning from the tissue in the left circular and right circular polarized states, respectively, as a function of depth d in the tissue. The light is initially in the left circularly polarized state at the surface of the tissue. Depolarization causes the light to be spread more equally between the two polarization states, pushing the degree of polarization towards 0. Birefringence causes the light to oscillate between the two states as a function of depth, causing banding where the degree of polarization varies from 1 to –1.

The PS-OCT system was also applied to detection of naturally occurring lesions in extracted human teeth. A cross-sectional PS-OCT image of a human tooth which contained visual indications of possible carious lesions is shown (fig. 14). Although the region of demineralized enamel is not clear in the backscattering intensity image (fig. 14, left), the polarization image (fig. 14, right) clearly shows demineralized enamel in the middle of the image with normal enamel above and below. The locations of demineralization were subsequently confirmed with histology. The vertical stripes visible at the top of

15

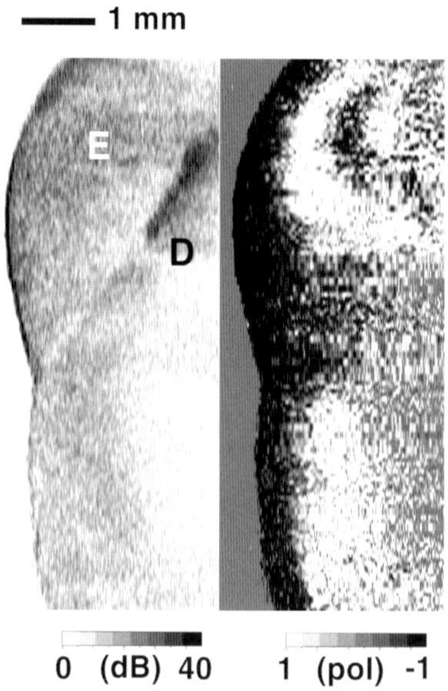

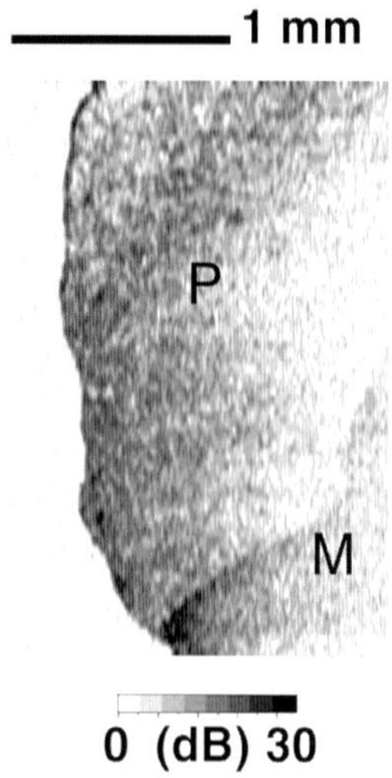

16

Fig. 15. Extracted tooth with caries occurring along the dentin/enamel interface. Contrary to demineralization in the enamel layer, caries that occurs in dentin is much easier to visualize in the OCT intensity plot (right) than in the OCT phase plot (left).

Fig. 16. In vivo OCT image of a porcelain crown and metal coping.

the crown (normal enamel) in the polarization image are caused by contour-dependent birefringence effects as described above.

Standard OCT systems, on the other hand, can be used to detect carious lesions in dentin [30]. We directly compared polarization and amplitude OCT images of a subsurface carious lesion along the DEJ to confirm this point (fig. 15). Unlike carious enamel, the carious dentin imaged was more easily seen in the backscattering intensity image (fig. 15, left) than in the polarization image (fig. 15, right). Since both intensity and polarization OCT provide useful information on the demineralization of carious lesions, future dental OCT systems will likely incorporate PS-OCT capabilities.

Restorations

A variety of restoration materials have also been imaged using dental OCT systems [13, 15]. The largest potential payoff of this effort is the ability to determine noninvasively the marginal and structural integrity of a given restoration. The most serious challenge to this effort is the limited imaging depths of existing OCT systems and their inability to penetrate metal copings. For example, shown here is an in vivo OCT image taken from the mid-facial

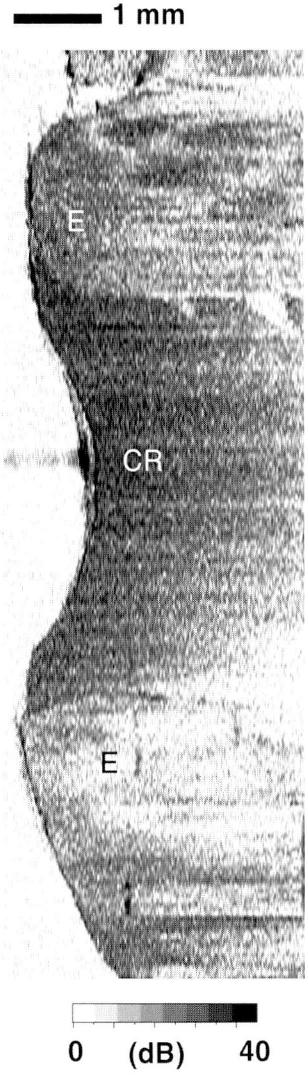

Fig. 17. In vivo OCT image, taken from the occlusal surface, of a composite restoration (middle).

tooth surface. The internal contours of a porcelain crown (P) are clearly visible here along with the metal coping (M) (fig. 16). The scattering properties of porcelain allow significant imaging depths to be obtained.

Other materials, such as composite restorations, have much higher scattering coefficients and therefore more limited imaging depths. Figure 17 is an in vivo OCT image taken from the occlusal surface. The composite material has a relatively unstructured scattering profile that is much denser than the adjoining enamel. The composite (CR), moreover, is not significantly birefringent compared to the surrounding enamel microstructure (E) as viewed from the occlusal surface of the tooth. This raises the potential of using birefringence artifacts as a contrast agent for discriminating the interface between the enamel and the restoration. These preliminary studies indicate OCT is potentially a powerful technique for visualizing structural and marginal restoration defects.

Perspectives

Prospects of OCT in Dentistry

The optical accessibility of clinically relevant structures in the oral cavity makes it a particularly attractive location to apply OCT imaging techniques. The periodontium, in particular, contains microstructures that are currently unresolvable with other noninvasive technologies. OCT is a potentially powerful tool for soft tissue diagnoses. Currently there are no cross-sectional imaging modalities that can be used intraorally for visualizing epithelial and connective tissue morphology.

OCT imaging could be used to identify demineralized enamel and dentinal caries. To determine the diagnostic efficacy of OCT for caries diagnoses, future studies targeted at correlating PS-OCT and OCT images of carious teeth with histological sectioning, along with patient-oriented clinical trials, are the logical next step towards validating this technique for caries detection. Finally, OCT could be used to evaluate the structural and marginal integrity of dental restorations. The most commonly used methods for evaluating the seal and structural integrity of restorations are visual and tactile examination [31, 32]. OCT will image and quantify marginal discrepancies with high resolution. The tomographic nature of the images should provide important information regarding the degree of mineralization of enamel of dental structure that is contiguous to the restoration margin. Further studies using extracted teeth are necessary to obtain a clear understanding of the limitations of OCT for this application.

Future Research for Dental OCT

Penetration depth and acquisition time must both be improved if OCT is to become a clinically useful technique. Brighter broadband light sources such as superluminescent diodes at 1.3 μm, fortunately, are becoming more widely available. This increase in the OCT incident sample power should significantly improve system dynamic range and allow real-time visualization of all periodontal regions, making the system clinically viable. It is also likely that future systems will trend towards PZT-modulated pathlength variation, since it offers the benefits of improved linearity, high-speed modulation and an absence of moving parts over current galvanometric scanning techniques. It is expected, finally, that alternative methods for improving image contrast, such as multiple wavelength OCT systems, could prove useful in dental applications.

References

1 Fujimoto J, DeDilvesti D, Ippen EP, Margolis R, Oseroff A: Femtosecond optical ranging in biological systems. Opt Lett 1996;11:150–152.

2 Benaron DA, Stevenson DK: Optical time-of-flight and absorbance imaging of biologic media. Science 1993;259:1463–1466.

3 Wang L, Ho PP, Liang X, Alfano RR: Kerr-Fourier imaging of hidden objects in thick turbid media. Opt Lett 1993;18:241–243.

4 Chen H, Chen Y, Dilworth D, Leith E, Lopez, J, Valdmanis J: Two-dimensional imaging through diffusing media using 150-fs gated electronic holography techniques. Opt Lett 1991;16:487–489.

5 Duncan MD: Time-gated imaging through scattering media using stimulated Raman amplification. Opt Lett 1991;16:1868–1870.

6 Hebden JC, Kruger RA, Wong S: Time resolved imaging through a highly scattering medium. Appl Opt 1991;30:788–794.

7 Youngquist RC, Carr S, Davies DEN: Optical coherence-domain reflectometry: A new optical evaluation technique. Opt Lett 1987;12:158–160.

8 Huang D, Swanson EA, Lin C, Shuman JS, Stinson W, Chang W, Hee MR, Flotte T, Gregory K, Puliafito CA, Fujimoto JG: Optical coherence tomography. Science 1991;254:1178–1181.

9 Hee MR, Puliafito CA, Wong C, Duker JS: Quantitative assessment of macular edema with optical coherence tomography. Arch Opthalmol 1995;113:1019–1029.

10 Schmidt JM, Yadlowsky MJ, Bonner RF: Subsurface imaging of living skin with optical coherence microscopy. Dermatology 1995;191:93–98.

11 Tearney GJ, Boppart SA, Bouma BE, Brezinski ME, Weissman NJ, Southern JF, Fujimoto JG: Scanning single-mode fiber optic catheter-endoscopic for optical coherence tomography. Opt Lett 1996;21:543–545.

12 Colston BW, Everett MJ, Da Silva LB, Otis LL, Stroeve P, Nathel H: Imaging of hard and soft tissue structure in the oral cavity by optical coherence tomography. Appl Opt 1998;37:3582–3585.

13 Colston BW, Sathyam US, Da Silva LB, Everett MJ, Stroeve P, Otis LL: Dental OCT. Opt Express 1998;3:230–238.

14 Baumgartenr A, Hitzenberger CK, Dichtl S, Sattmann H, Moritz A, Sperr W, Fercher AF: Optical coherence tomography of dental structures. SPIE 1998;3248:130–136.

15 Feldchtein FI, Gelikonov GV, Gelikonov VM, Iksanov RR, Kuranov RV, Sergeev AM, Gladkova ND, Ourutina MN, Warren JA, Reitze DH: In vivo OCT imaging of hard and soft tissue of the oral cavity. Opt Express 1998;3:239–250.

16 Mayfield L, Bratthall G, Attstrom R: Periodontal probe precision using four different periodontal probes. J Clin Periodontol 1996;23:76–82.

17 Pihlstrom BL: Measurement of attachment level in clinical trails – Probing methods. J Periodontol 1992;63:1072–1077.

18 Hintze H, Wenzel A, Larsen MJ: Steromicroscopy, film radiography, microradiography and naked-eye inspection of tooth sections as validation for occlusal caries diagnosis. Caries Res 1995;29:359–363.

19 Wenzel A: Digital radiography and caries diagnosis. Dentomaxillofac Radiol 1998;1:3–11.

20 Mandel L, Wolf E: Optical coherence and Quantum Optics. Cambridge, Cambridge University Press, 1995.
21 Born M, Wolf E: Principles of Optics. New York, Pergamon Press, 1993.
22 Haus H: Waves and Fields in Optoelectronics. Englewood Cliffs, Prentice-Hall, 1984.
23 Welch A, van Gemert M (eds): Optical-Thermal Response of Laser-Irradiated Tissue. Lasers, Photonics, and Electro-Optics. New York, Plenum Press, 1995.
24 Hee MR, Izatt JA, Swanson EA, Fujimoto JG: Femtosecond transillumination tomography in thick tissues. Opt Lett 1993;18:1107–1109.
25 Van de Hulst HC: Light Scattering by Small Particles. New York, Dover, 1987.
26 Palmer KF, Williams D: Optical properties of water in the near infrared. J Opt Soc Am 1974;64: 1107–1110.
27 Parsa P, Jacques SL, Nishioka NS: Optical properties of rat liver between 350 and 2,200 nm. Appl Opt 1989;28:2325–2330.
28 Fried D, Glena RE, Featherstone JD, Seka W: Nature of light scattering in dental enamel and dentin at visible an near-infrared wavelengths. Appl Opt 1995;34:1278–1285.
29 Everett MJ, Colston BW Jr, Sathyam US, Da Silva LB, Fried JD, Featherstone JD: Non-invasive diagnosis of early caries with polarization sensitive optical coherence tomography (PS-OCT). SPIE. Proc Lasers in Dentistry V, 1999, vol 3593.
30 Warren JA, Gelikonov GV, Feldchtein FI, Sergeev AM, Beach NM, Moores MD, Reitze DH: Imaging and characterization of dental structure using optical coherence tomography. Opt Soc Am Techn Digest 1998;6:128.
31 Cvar JF, Ryge G: Criteria for the Clinical Evaluation of Dental Restoration Materials. San Francisco, US Dept HEW PHS, Dental Health Center, 1971.
32 Moss-Salentijn L, Hendricks-Klyvert M: Dental and Oral Tissues. Philadelphia, Lea & Febiger, 1990.

Bill Colston, Lawrence Livermore National Laboratory,
7000 East Avenue, L-399, Livermore, CA 94550 (USA)
Tel. +1 925 423 0375, Fax +1 925 424 2778, E-Mail Colston1@llnl.gov

Faller RV (ed): Assessment of Oral Health.
Monogr Oral Sci. Basel, Karger, 2000, vol 17, pp 56–72

Advances in Measurements of Periodontal Bone and Attachment Loss

Marjorie K. Jeffcoat, Michael S. Reddy

Department of Periodontics, University of Alabama School of Dentistry, Birmingham, Ala., USA

Abstract

Periodontal probing and measurements using intraoral radiographs are widely utilized clinical techniques to measure attachment and bone levels, respectively. Determination of progressive disease, healing, or regeneration in clinical studies may require maximal sensitivity and attention to measurement error in order to assure that changes detected by new methodology are accurate. Both types of methods are susceptible to errors due to resolution, repeatability, and accuracy of the technique. While both probing and radiographic methods are useful in clinical trials they vary widely with respect to these errors. For example, manual probing is repeatable to within 1 mm better than 90% of the time, and state-of-the-art radiographic methods, such as digital subtraction radiography, can detect as little as 1 mg of bony change.

Assessment of periodontal disease routinely utilizes physical inspection and examination, periodontal probing, and radiographs. These assessments are used to quantify two strikingly different measures of periodontitis. The first is the extent and severity of existing periodontitis and the second is the progression of periodontitis.

Extent and Severity of Existing Periodontitis

The extent and severity of existing periodontitis represents the sum total of disease and healing of the lifespan of a tooth [1]. For example, a tooth surface which exhibits 5 mm of attachment loss may have lost the attachment over several decades, over the past year, or may have previously exhibited 8 mm of attachment loss and been treated in order to regain attachment. Measures of the extent and severity are taken at a single point in time during one examination. In research, these variables are frequently used for cross-sectional and epidemiologic studies, or as baseline measurements for longitudinal studies.

Probing depth, frequently measured in clinical practice, is a measure of the distance (in millimeters) from the gingival margin to the clinical attachment which is the position where resistance is met by the probe at the base of the pocket. The clinical attachment level (CAL) is the distance from a fixed landmark on the tooth, such as the cemento-enamel junction (CEJ), to the pocket base. Relative attachment loss may also be measured using a landmark on the tooth or a removable reference such as a stent. Since these relative measures are not necessarily related to root length, they are not useful to measure the severity of disease in a single examination because the location of the landmark is arbitrary. Relative measures of attachment levels are, however, useful for sequential measurements for the calculation of the progression of attachment loss over time.

Diagnostic Assessment: Resolution, Repeatability and Accuracy

Much of the literature uses different terms, therefore it is worthwhile to define these measures before proceeding to discuss their influence on periodontal diagnosis.

Resolution relates to the smallest change in the measured value to which an instrument will respond. At times this quality is referred to as precision in the periodontal literature.

Repeatability refers to the ability of the method to obtain the same answer when the test is performed more than once. Repeatability may refer to intraoperator or interoperator repeatability.

Accuracy is the closeness with which the reading of an instrument approaches the true value of the variable being measured. In the periodontal literature this quality is also referred to as bias or validity. Diagnostic accuracy is assessed in terms of sensitivity and specificity. The use of this paradigm is predicted on a knowledge of the state of the disease. Sensitivity is a measure of the ability of a test to detect disease when it is present. Specificity is a measure of the ability to rule out disease when it is absent.

Each of these measures are important descriptors of a physical test for periodontal disease. But any single descriptor does not fully describe the performance of the test in a clinical situation. For example, a hypothetical periodontal probe that can measure to 0.01 mm (high resolution, indeed), but

Table 1. Reproducibility of clinical attachment levels within 1 mm

Measurement	Reproducibility, %	Reference
CAL	94.8	5
CAL	94.5	6
CAL	93.9	7
CAL	77–84	8
RAL	90–91	8
CAL	93–95	9
CAL	98.8–82.6	10
RAL	94.1–97.5	11

CAL = Clinical attachment level; RAL = relative attachment level.

is repeatable only to the nearest millimeter, may be no better than a conventional probe for the diagnosis of periodontal disease.

Periodontal Probing

Resolution

Periodontal probing is a fundamental part of the intraoral examination and the need for improved resolution in periodontal probes has long been recognized. The markings on the conventional probe are spaced at 1, 2 or 3 mm resulting in a resolution of 1 mm (or 0.5 mm if interpolation by the examiner using a probe marked in millimeters is used). Electronic probes represent an improvement over the resolution of the conventional periodontal probe. For example, the Florida probe [2], as well as prototype probes under study at the University of Alabama [3] and at the University of Toronto have resolutions of 0.1 mm [4].

Repeatability

Improved resolution does not always translate into improved repeatability of measurement. Resolution simply quantifies the ability of the electronics to detect a change in depth. This is a function of the design of the instrument while repeatability is greatly influenced by the operator's use of the instrument. Variations in instrument angulation and the consistency of probing force will seriously influence the repeatability of measurement, while having no effect on

Table 2. Comparison of repeatability of conventional and force controlled probes

Comparison	Result	Reference
Florida probe vs. conventional probe	Repeatability (SD) Conventional probe 0.81 mm Florida probe single pass 1.15 mm Florida double pass 0.44 mm	9
Florida probe vs. conventional probe	Conventional probe 0.62 mm Florida probe single pass 0.82 mm Florida probe double pass 0.63 mm	12
Florida probe vs. conventional probe	Conventional probe 0.84 mm Florida probe single pass 0.59 mm	13
Modified Florida vs. conventional probe	Conventional probe 0.39 mm Florida probe single pass 0.62 mm	14

SD = Standard deviation of the difference of duplicate measurements (used as an index of repeatability); single pass = a single measurement taken at each site is used as the measurement; double pass = two measurements are taken at each site, the measurements may be averaged and/or a third measurement taken if the variability exceeds the investigator-defined threshold.

the probe's resolution. Table 1 compares the repeatability of probing methods without the use of force controlled probes. A high degree of repeatability within 1 mm of error was observed across studies.

Table 2 compares the repeatability of manual and force controlled probes. Osborn et al. [9, 12] compared the repeatability error in determining the probing attachment level relative to a fixed landmark obtained using the manual Michigan O probe and the Florida disk probe. The Michigan O probe was used to make measurements of attachment loss relative to the CEJ with a resolution of 1.0 mm. The Florida disk probe is a controlled force periodontal probe that is capable of measuring the probing attachment level relative to the occlusal surface of the tooth with a resolution of 0.1 mm. It should be remembered that measurements of the probing attachment level relative to the occlusal surface are not meaningful indicators of the severity of destruction since the measurement incorporates the tooth height in the measurement. Therefore, the Florida disk probe is used to obtain measurements over time which may be compared to determine whether or not a site has evidence of progressive probing attachment loss. The investigators reported that if each site is measured once during each examination, use of the electronic probe offered no advantage over the conventional probe in reducing examiner error. However, if the same examiner measured each site twice in order to identify and correct gross probing errors of >1 mm, use of the Florida disk probe significantly reduced the repeatability error.

Reddy et al. [14] compared the repeatability of conventional probing measured to 1 or 0.5 mm and force controlled probing measured relative to a stent. Both conventional and controlled force probes resulted in intra- and interoperator repeatability of better than 0.9 mm. No significant advantage was offered by the electronic probe.

In an excellent review, Armitage [15] presented a comprehensive summary of the evidence base underlying periodontal diagnosis. This was used for consensus development as part of the 1996 World Workshop in Periodontology. The consensus report found there was no advantage to force controlled probes except for the convenience of automatic recording.

Voice recognition has been used as an alternate method for automatic recording. Custom software may facilitate automatic recording and comparison of examination. A recent study has shown that specially developed systems which accommodate different accents are better than 99% accurate [16].

These findings have important potential implications for clinical trials and for the role of electronic probes in periodontal practice. By itself, an improvement in resolution did not necessarily result in improved repeatability because the increased resolution provides more opportunities for measurements to disagree. Care must also be exercised when using multiple measurements to 'correct' for errors and then using those data to describe instrument repeatability. The investigator can create almost any desired level of repeatability by repeating the measurements until the desired level of repeatability is achieved. This caution applies to the comparison of repeatability data across probes and methods, but should not be taken to say correction of gross errors in the clinical situation according to a fixed protocol is inappropriate.

Accuracy

Accuracy data are critical because a method may be repeatable but incorrect. Unfortunately, the periodontal literature is relatively sparse with respect to accuracy or validity studies for the new periodontal probing methods. This is likely due to the fact that the gold standard for CAL is histology and histology is by definition a destructive and invasive technique. Nonetheless, two sources of error, probing force and extent of gingival inflammation, have been shown to influence probing accuracy (table 3).

The effect of gingival inflammation per se on probing measurements is also a source of accuracy error. In now classic papers, Magnusson and List-

Table 3. Accuracy of clinical attachment levels determined using probes

Study type	Accuracy	Force	Reference
Case-control study in patients	Treated patients −0.73 mm Untreated patients +0.45 mm	0.5 N Force 0.5 N Force	17
Beagles	Healthy beagles −0.39 mm Experimental gingivitis −0.10 mm PD +0.24 mm	25 g 25 g 25 g	18
Beagles	Gingivitis −0.84 mm PD with moderate inflammation −0.05 mm PD with severe inflammation +0.50 mm	Undefined Undefined Undefined	19
Case-control study in patients	Probe penetration increases linearly with GI Probe penetration tended to increase with force	20–30 g	20
Non-controlled cases with severe periodontitis	Probe penetration increases with increasing insertion force	0.5–1.25 N	21
Case-control study in patients	PD ≥4 mm untreated +0.29 mm PD ≥4 mm treated −0.31 mm PD ≤3 mm untreated −0.01 mm PD ≤3 mm treated +0.02 mm	Metal strips used as probes	22, 23
Florida probe case-controlled	Controlled force probe under measured relative to conventional relative to conventional probe Controlled force −0.48 mm Conventional probe +0.08 mm		24

GI = Gingival inflammation; PD = peridontitis.

garten [22] demonstrated that the probe may penetrate an average of 0.29 mm into inflamed tissue while remaining an average of 0.31 mm coronal to the connective tissue attachment in non-inflamed tissue. Garnick et al. [25] reexamined the effects of inflammation, probing pressure, and probe displacement in gingivitis in beagles. The location of the probe tip is both clinically and histologically related to probing pressure and that selection of the appropriate pressure can result in measurements at the base of the crevice or at the connective tissue attachment. Not surprisingly, the authors found that the pressure needed to probe to the base of the crevice was less than the pressure needed to probe to the connective tissue attachment. The reader should note one important difference between this recent paper and papers in the older literature. The article by Garnick et al. [25] refers to probing pressure while the older papers refer to probing force. The pressure delivered at the base of the pocket is determined by both probing force and tip design. Thus, two instruments may use the same probing force but deliver very different pressures to the base of the pocket.

Other studies have compared CAL measurements taken using force controlled probes with measurements obtained using conventional manual probes (table 3). Available force controlled instruments underestimate the CAL relative to conventional probing.

Assessment of Disease Progression

Disease progression is traditionally determined from repeated examinations over time. Progression is calculated as the difference in probing attachment levels during a given time period. Since errors in measurements are additive, calculation of progression requires optimal repeatability and accuracy.

Many studies have examined the ability of a single measure of probing (bone loss or other clinical indicator, such as bleeding on probing) to predict disease progression (table 4). In these studies, the gold standard for progressive disease was sequential examination. The preponderance of the evidence indicates that a single measure of the CAL is highly specific in ruling out progressive periodontitis [15]. Interestingly a single measure provides little sensitivity in predicting progressive periodontitis [15]. In other words, sites which do not have disease based on a single examination are unlikely to undergo a progressive CAL, while sites with an existing CAL may or may not undergo progressive clinical attachment loss.

Effects of Measurement on the Prevalence of Active Disease

Measurement accuracy and repeatability influences our perception of the prevalence of active attachment loss. Investigators have long recognized the need to assess measurement error and to consider sites which exhibit progressive clinical attachment loss above the measurement error as active sites. In now classic studies, a 3-mm threshold for change in CALs between examination was used. These studies reported a low prevalence of disease activity of 5–7%.

Table 4. Clinical parameters and progression of periodontitis

Parameter	Sensitivity	Specificity	Treatment	Reference
Redness	0.32	0.74	Untreated	26
Redness	0.57	0.46	Untreated	27
Suppuration	0.01	1.00	Treated	28
Suppuration	0.19	0.98	Treated	29
Suppuration	0.38	0.86	Untreated	30
Suppuration	0.05	0.98	Treated	31
BOP at 4/4 visits	0.20	0.97	Treated	32
BOP at 2/4 visits	0.83	0.50	Treated	32
BOP at 8/8 visits	0.15	0.88	Treated	28
BOP 5/9 visits	0.47	0.84	Treated no maintenance	29
BOP 7/9 visits	0.45	0.96	Treated no maintenance	29
Meta-analysis of BOP	0.44	0.76		15
PD $\leq$3 mm	0.69	0.25	Untreated	26
PD 4–6 mm	0.21	0.84	Untreated	26
PD $\geq$7	0.12	0.92	Untreated	26
PD $\leq$3 mm	0.47	0.26	Untreated	27
PD 4–5.9	0.28	0.82	Untreated	27
PD $\geq$6	0.26	0.89	Untreated	27
PD $\geq$5 mm	0.93	0.08	Untreated	30

BOP = Bleeding on probing, PD = periodontitis.

When a high-accuracy, high-resolution probe is used, disease activity may appear up to 6 times more prevalent than when a conventional probe is used [1, 33–35]. The detection of active sites will be influenced by the analytic method used to detect changes [36].

Radiographic Methods

A continuum of radiographic methods exist which have different levels of method resolution, repeatability and accuracy [37, 38]. Radiographs are used to assess bone support in one of three major ways. These include interpretation of the radiographic image, measurement and image processing. The accuracy and repeatability of the radiographic methods are summarized in table 5. Interpretation of the radiographic image, by transillumination on a view-box, is of course, the most frequently used method in clinical practice

Table 5. Accuracy and repeatability of radiographic methods for assessment of bone loss

Measurement	Result	Reference
Bone height	Repeatable to 0.08 mm using geometric correction	39, 40
	Repeatable to 0.5 mm using nonstandardized films	41, 42
Bone loss as a percent of root length	Repeatable to 2.7%	40, 43
	Repeatable to 1.47%	
Digital subtraction radiography		
Detection of change	Able to detect bone changes difficult to see by eye	44, 45, 46
	Detect 1–5% change by ^{125}I absorptiometry with high sensitivity	47
	Detects 1 mg change with 87.8% sensitivity and 100% specificity	62
Measurement of mass	Correlation between actual and measured mass of >94%	62
Measurement of density	Correlation between actual and measured density of >94%	48, 49

today. Measurements taken from the radiograph allow quantification of the extent of bone loss along the root surface and may utilize very simple methods such as a grid or Schei ruler [50], or may use state-of-the-art computerized techniques [28, 44, 51, 52]. Digital radiography is especially useful to detect small changes in hard tissues which occur between examinations. Image-processing techniques, such as subtraction radiography, are primarily used in research, and exploit information contained in the radiograph that is too subtle to be seen by eye. In brief, the purpose of digital subtraction radiography (DSR) is to subtract all unchanging structures from a set of two X-ray films displaying only the area of change. The image-processing procedure subtracts unchanging teeth, cortical bone, and trabecular pattern leaving only the bone gain or loss standing out against a neutral gray background on the subtraction image.

A single radiograph will only yield information regarding evidence of past episodes of disease activity and healing. Thus, interpretation of the single radiograph provides the clinician with information analogous to the single probing examination and is best suited to screening for the presence of periodontitis. Many now classic studies have shown that interpretive radiology only detects changes in bone after 30–50% of the bone mineral has been lost. Errors in film geometry and processing, and the ability of the practitioner to interpret the film also strongly limit the repeatability of interpretive radiology [38, 53].

In order to detect active bone loss over time, two or more radiographic examinations must be compared. As in the comparison of probing attachment level measurements, the issues of method resolution, repeatability and accuracy come into play.

Resolution

Resolution becomes an issue for measurement and image-processing methods to assess the severity and progression of bone loss. The simplest methods for the quantitative assessment of alveolar bone loss involve direct measurements from the CEJ to the alveolar bone level on radiographs. The resolution of this method may vary from 1 mm when a ruler is used on a conventional film, to approximately 0.05 mm when an image-processing system is used to enlarge the radiograph and measure the bone height [39, 40]. The Schei ruler technique expresses bone height as a percent of root length [50]. The resolution of this method depends on the number of spokes used in the Schei ruler. Generally, this methodology can resolve 10–20% bone loss.

Repeatability

There are limited studies concerning the repeatability of bone height measurements. In early studies, Jeffcoat et al. [39] assessed the repeatability of the Schei ruler or the percent alveolar bone loss from radiographs of beagles with periodontitis. Calibration data taken over a 3-year period in our laboratory revealed less than 0.5-mm error using vertical bite-wing radiographs in patients with moderate periodontitis. Similar data have been reported by Hausmann et al. [41, 42, 54, 55] who recommended this use of the bite-wing radiograph and promulgated the need for rules for the investigator to utilize in order to minimize errors.

Albander [56] assessed the repeatability and accuracy of CEJ-to-crest measurements on standardized and non-standardized periapical films in relation to direct measurements on skulls. Excellent correlations (98–99%) between measurements made with both radiographic measures were observed, but both methods tended to underestimate proximal bone loss. It should be noted that in this study the authors enlarged the radiographs, but made direct measurements on the skulls. Therefore, the resolution of the measurements from enlarged radiographic measurements was 0.01 mm, but only 0.1 mm for direct measurements.

In data derived from a regeneration study, Matsuda et al. [57] were able to correlate bone loss (CEJ to infrabony defect base) on vertical bite-wing radiographs, as well as clinical measurements of attachment loss with direct bone loss measurements obtained during surgery. Significant correlations were observed.

Image-processing techniques, such as DSR, are used to detect and measure the progression of bone loss between sequential radiographic examinations. The DSR system has several components of repeatability error. It is the need for excellent repeatability that makes the performance of subtraction radiography particularly technique-sensitive. In order to subtract radiographs, they must be taken with nearly identical angulation, contrast, and density. Geometry may be standardized either with custom positioning devices [53] or using a cephalostat, and residual errors corrected with computer software [58]. Excellent methods have been developed which use software to correct for the source of repeatability error due to differences in film contrast and density [59]. Algorithms which color areas of bone loss, gain and no change in different colors, have been shown to improve the agreement among investigators and enhance the ability of novice clinicians to detect changes with DSR [60, 61].

The accuracy of the subtraction method to detect small osseous changes has been validated by several investigators by comparing the ability of clinicians to detect small simulated lesions on conventional radiographs and on subtraction images. The clinicians were unable to detect defects of $<5\%$ bone loss on pairs of conventional radiographs with any better probability than chance. Use of subtraction imaging techniques allowed the observers to detect or rule out the presence of these tiny lesions with a sensitivity and specificity of better than 90% [23, 53, 62, 63].

For the long term, the power of radiographic image processing for dentistry lies not only in the ability to detect a small lesion, but in the ability to detect and size that lesion in terms of length, area, volume and mass of bone loss or gain. To perform this task, specialized software is needed to detect the lesion and determine its size. The thickness of bone loss or gain may be estimated by further analyzing the gray levels in subtraction radiographs, and relating the gray levels in the region of change to a reference wedge contained in the radiograph [62]. The use of quantitative methodology has been introduced with computer-assisted densitometric image analysis [64], which has been used to study remodeling following periodontal surgery in interproximal and furcation sites.

Such methods are currently the state-of-the-art for dental image processing. The accuracy of such methods are currently undergoing evaluation. However, additional sources of accuracy error are present for these quantitative radiographic techniques. These include localization and sizing of the lesion and beam hardening errors [65]. Computer algorithms and radiographic techniques are presently in use and under development which limit these sources of error and can detect and size lesions with as little as 3–5% accuracy error [66].

Table 6. Relationship between radiographic and clinical attachment level changes

Type of study	Comparison	Concordance	Reference
Longitudinal	Adult periodontitis	75.8%	67
Longitudinal	Adult periodontitis	82%	68
Longitudinal	Adult periodontitis Healthy patients	77.1%	69
Longitudinal	Adult periodontitis	80.4%	35
Longitudinal	Adult periodontitis	Not explicitly stated but high degree not observed	30
Case study	Adult periodontitis	Correlation between distance from CEJ to bone crest vs. clinical attachment level = 0.80	70

CEJ = Cemento-enamel junction.

Errors due to image processing and measurement also contribute to total system errors. Most articles have expressed total system error rather than individually measuring each potential component of error. The system repeatability of DSR has been measured in vitro using skulls, and in vivo in monkeys using simulated feather-edged osseous lesions fabricated of bone-equivalent material. Intraoperator repeatability was better than 90% and there was no significant difference in repeatability between operators [63].

The ability of radiographs exposed in a multicenter study to detect small osseous changes using DSR in human subjects has been reported. Lesions were simulated using small feather-edged hydroxyapatite chips (approximately 1, 7, and 10 mg). The overall sensitivity and specificity in detecting 1-mg changes was 87.8 and 100%, respectively. The sensitivity and specificity in detecting 7- and 10-mg chips was 100%. A strong linear relationship between actual lesion mass was observed ($R^2 = 0.94$, slope = 0.98, $p < 0.0001$). No significant differences were observed by center [62].

Relationship Between Radiographic Evidence of Bone Loss and Changes in Probing Attachment Levels

The relationship between changes in probing attachment levels and alveolar bone changes remains somewhat controversial. Pertinent studies describing the degree of concordance of the two methods are shown in table 6. The highest degree of concordance is achieved when measurement methods of similar accuracy and resolution are utilized in untreated patients. As the tissue tone changes as a result of periodontal therapy, larger changes may be observed in the clinical attachment measurements than in bone measurements.

In a recently completed study by Reddy et al. [67], the progression of bone and clinical attachment loss over an 18-month period in 40 patients with moderate periodontitis were compared. Patients were untreated except for supragingival prophylaxes performed every 3 months. The relative CAL was measured monthly relative to a stent using a previously described modified Florida probe. Sites with progression of bone loss were identified by significant slopes of the regression line of attachment loss versus time. Standardized radiographs were exposed at 6-month intervals for quantitative DSR. Specialized software was used to measure changes in bone support that occurred during the 18-month study period in millimeters along the root surfaces.

New data from this study are presented here. On an individual site basis, there was a significant increase in the progression of clinical attachment loss with an increasing progression of bone loss ($p < 0.000001$). Sites that exhibited no bone loss by subtraction radiography had a mean progression of CAL of 0.72 ± 0.16 mm, while sites with progressive bone loss had significantly higher progression of CAL of 2.16 ± 0.19 mm ($p < 0.000001$). Mean progression tended to be higher when assessed using CAL measurements than with radiographic imaging. When attachment loss is taken as the standard, the sensitivity of DSR in detecting progression of CAL was 70.6%, while its ability to rule out progressive CAL was 86.2%. On a site basis, the overall concordance between progressive bone loss and CAL was 75.8%. These data indicate a clear association between progression of periodontitis as measured by CAL using an electronic probe, and alveolar bone loss as measured by quantitative DSR.

Other investigators have shown similar results (table 6). Other studies did not have a high degree of concordance [29]. Most frequently these studies utilized radiographic and CAL measurements with very different levels of repeatability and accuracy or also reflected changes in tissue inflammation following therapy.

Conclusions

Both periodontal probing and measurements from radiographs can provide standards for assessment of corrective tissue attachment loss and alveolar bone loss, respectively. If a single type of examination is to be used, selection will be dependent on the hypothesis to be tested (i.e. effect on connective tissue or bone). Further selection of the specific type of probing or radiographic technique will be dependent on the balance between resolution, repeatability and accuracy, in addition to the amount of time and cost required to perform the examination.

For the future, automated examinations that include voice recording of the examination and measurements of progressive loss of bone height will be facilitated by continued development of accurate direct digital radiograph machines. Such machines have the potential to eliminate the digitization step when using conventional radiographs and to reduce patient radiation exposure by 80–90%.

Eventually, the end result may permit rapid assessment of progressive periodontitis. On-going research will improve these techniques and preliminary data have shown a moderately high correlation between oral and systemic bone loss.

References

1 Jeffcoat M, Reddy MD: Detection of periodontal disease activity: Comparison of probing and subtraction radiography (abstract 270). J Dent Res 1990:69:142.

2 Gibbs CH, Hirschfeld JW, Lee JG, Low SB, Magnusson I, Thousand RR, Yermini P, Clark WB: Description and clinical evaluation of a new computerized periodontal probe – The Florida probe. J Clin Periodontol 1988;15:137–144.

3 Jeffcoat MK, Jeffcoat R, Captain K: A periodontal probe with automated cemento-enamel junction detection-design and clinical trials. IEEE Trans Biomed Eng 1991;38:330–333.

4 Birek P, McCulloch CAG, Hardy V: Gingival attachment level measurements with an automated periodontal probe. J Clin Periodontol 1987;14:472–477.

5 Glavind L, Löe H: Errors in the clinical assessment of periodontal destruction. J Periodont Res 1967;2:179–184.

6 Smith L, Suomi J, Greene J, Barbano J: A study of intra-examiner variation in scoring oral hygiene status, gingival inflammation and epithelial attachment level. J Periodontol 1970;41:671–674.

7 Isidor F, Karring T, Attström R: Reproducibility of pocket depth and attachment level measurements when using a flexible splint. J Clin Periodontol 1984;11:662–668.

8 Badersten A, Nilveus R, Egelberg J: Reproducibility of probing attachment level measurements. J Clin Periodontol 1984;11:475–485.

9 Osborn J, Stoltenberg J, Huso B, Aeppli D, Pihlstrom B: Comparison of measurement variability using a standard and constant force periodontal probe. J Periodontol 1990;61(suppl):497–503.

10 Kingman A, Löe H, Anerud A, Boysen H: Errors in measuring parameters associated with periodontal health disease. J Periodontol 1991;62:477–486.

11 Wang S-F, Leknes K, Zimmerman G, Sigurdsson T, Wikesjö U, Selvig K: Reproducibility of periodontal probing using a conventional manual and an automated force-controlled electronic probe. J Periodontol 1995;66:38–46.

12 Osborn JB, Stoltenberg JL, Huso BA, Aeppli DM, Pihlstrom BL: Comparison of measurement variability in subjects with moderate periodontitis using a conventional and constant force periodontal probe. J Periodontol 1992;62:283–289.

13 Rams TE, Slots J: Comparison of two pressure sensitive probes and a manual periodontal probe in shallow and deep pockets. Int J Periodontics Restorative Dent 1993;13:521–529.

14 Reddy MS, Palcanis K, Geurs N: Comparison of manual and controlled force periodontal probing. J Dent Res 1995;74:1302.

15 Armitage GC: Periodontal diseases: Diagnosis. Ann Periodontol 1996;1:37–215.

16 Ramp L, Geurs N, Ramp M, Jeffcoat RL: Performance of computer speech recognition for clinical data recording. J Dent Res 1999 (special issue): in press.
17 Fowler C, Garrett S, Crigger M, Egelberg J: Histologic probe position in treated and untreated human periodontal tissues. J Clin Periodontol 1982;9:373–385.
18 Armitage GC, Svanberg CK, Löe H: Microscopic evaluation of clinical measurements of connective tissue attachment levels. J Clin Periodontol 1977;4:173–190.
19 Jansen J, Pilot T, Corba N: Histologic evaluation of probe penetration during clinical assessment of periodontal attachment levels. An investigation of experimentally induced periodontal lesions in beagle dogs. J Clin Periodontol 1981;8:98–106.
20 Robinson PJ, Vitek RM: The relationship between gingival inflammation and resistance to probe penetration. J Periodont Res 1979;14:185–268.
21 van der Velden U: Probing force and the relationship of the probe tip to the periodontal tissues. J Clin Periodontol 1979;6:106–114.
22 Magnusson I, Listgarten MA: Histological evaluation of probing depth following periodontal treatment. J Clin Periodont 1980;7:26–31.
23 Listgarten MA: Periodontal probing: What does it mean? J Clin Periodontol 1980:7:165–175.
24 Hull PS, Clerehugh V, Ghassemi-Aval A: An assessment of the validity of a constant force electronic probe in measuring probing depths. J Periodontol 1995;66:848–851.
25 Garnick JJ, Keagle JG, Searle JR, King GE, Thompson WO: Gingival resistance to probing forces. II. The effect of inflammation and pressure on probe displacement in beagle dog gingivitis. J Periodontol 1989:60:498–505.
26 Haffajee AD, Socransky SS, Goodson JM: Comparison of different data analyses for detecting changes in attachment level. J Clin Periodontol 1983;10:298–310.
27 Halazonetis T, Haffajee A, Socransky S: Relationship of clinical parameters to attachment loss in subsets of subjects with destructive periodontal diseases. J Clin Periodontol 1989;16:563–568.
28 Kaldahl WB, Kalkwarf KL, Patil KD, Molvar MP: Relationship of gingival bleeding, gingival suppuration, and supragingival plaque to attachment loss. J Periodontol 1990;61:347–351.
29 Badersten A, Nilveus R, Egelberg J: Effect of nonsurgical periodontal therapy. VII. Bleeding, suppuration and probing depth in sites with probing attachment loss. J Clin Periodontol 1985;12: 432–440.
30 Armitage GC, Jeffcoat MK, Chadwick DE, Taggart EJ, Numabe Y, Landis JR, Weaver SL, Sharp TJ: Longitudinal evaluation of elastase as a marker for the progression of periodontitis. J Periodontol 1994;65:120–128.
31 Magnusson I, Marks R, Clark W, Walker C, Low S, McArthur W: Clinical microbiological and immunological characteristics of subjects with 'refractory' periodontal disease. J Clin Periodontol 1991;18:291–299.
32 Lang NP, Nyman S, Senn C, Joss A: Bleeding on probing as it relates to probing pressure and gingival health. J Clin Periodontol 1991;18:257–261.
33 Jeffcoat MK, Reddy MS: Progression of probing attachment loss in adult periodontitis. J Periodontol 1991;62:185–189.
34 Armitage GC, Jeffcoat MK, Chadwick DE, Taggart EJ, Numabo Y, Landis JR, Weaver SL, Sharp TJ: Evaluation of elastase in the progression of periodontitis. J Periodontol 1994;65:120–128.
35 Palcanis K, Larjava I, Wells B, Suggs K, Jeffcoat M: Elastase as an indicator of periodontal disease progression. J Periodontol 1992;63:237–242.
36 Aeppli DM, Philstrom BL: Detection of longitudinal change in periodontitis. J Periodont Res 1989; 5:329–334.
37 Hausmann E: A contemporary perspective on techniques for the clinical assessment of alveolar bone. J Periodontol 1990;61:149–156.
38 Jeffcoat MK, Wang I-C, Reddy MS: Radiographic diagnosis in periodontitis. Periodontol 2000 1995;7:54–68.
39 Jeffcoat MK, Williams RC: Relationship between linear and area measurements of radiographic bone levels using simple computerized techniques. J Periodontol Res 1984;19:191–198.
40 Jeffcoat MK, Jeffcoat R, Williams RC: A new method for the comparison of bone loss measurements on non-standardized radiographs. J Periodont Res 1984;19:434–440.

41 Hausmann E, Allen K, Christersson L, Genco RJ: Effect of x-ray beam vertical angulation on radiographic alveolar crest level measurement. J Periodont Res 1989;24:8–19.
42 Hausmann E, Allen K, Dunford R, Christersson L: A reliable computerized method to determine the level of the radiographic alveolar crest. J Periodont Res 1989;24:368–369.
43 Jeffcoat MK, Williams RC, Kaplan ML, Goldhaber P: Bone-seeking radiopharmaceutical uptake as an indicator of active alveolar bone loss in untreated and surgically treated teeth in beagle dogs. J Periodont Res 1985;20:307–316.
44 Webber RL, Ruttiman UE, Grondahl HG: X-ray image subtraction as a basis for assessment of periodontal changes. J Periodont Res 1982;17:509–511.
45 Grondahl HG, Grondahl K: Subtraction radiography for the diagnosis of periodontal bone lesions. Oral Surg Oral Med Oral Pathol 1983;55:208–213.
46 Braegger U, Litch J, Pasquali L, Kornman KS: Computer assisted densitometric image analysis for the quantitation of radiographic alveolar bone changes. J Periodont Res 1987;22:227–229.
47 Ortman LF, Dunford R, McHenry K, Hausmann E: Subtraction radiography and computer assisted densitometric analyses of standardized radiographs. A comparison study with 125 I absorptiometry. J Periodont Res 1985;20:644–651.
48 Reddy MS, Weatherford TW, Smith CA, West BD, Jeffcoat MK, Jacks TM: Alendronate treatment of naturally occurring periodontitis in beagles. J Periodontol 1995;66:211–217.
49 Jeffcoat MK, Reddy MS: Alveolar bone loss and osteoporosis: Evidence for a common mode of therapy using the bisphonate alendronate; in Davidovitch Z (eds): The Biologic Mechanism of Tooth Resorption and Replacement by Implants. Boston, Harvard Society for the Advancement of Orthodontics, 1996, pp 365–373.
50 Schei O, Waerhaug J, Lovdal A, Arno A: Alveolar bone loss as related to oral hygiene and age. J Periodontol 1959;30:7–16.
51 Grondahl K, Kullendorff B, Strid KG, Grondahl HG, Henrikson CO: Detectability of artificial marginal bone lesions as a function of lesion depth. A comparison between subtraction radiography and conventional radiographic technique. J Clin Periodontol 1988;15:156–162.
52 Brägger U, Pasquali L, Weber H, Kornman KS: Computer-assisted densitometric image analysis (CADIA) for the assessment of alveolar bone density changes in furcations. J Clin Periodontol 1989;16:46–52.
53 Hausmann E, Christersson L, Dunford R, Wikesjo U, Phyo J, Genco RJ: Usefulness of subtraction radiography in the evaluation of periodontal therapy. J Periodontol 1985;56:4–7.
54 Hausmann E, Allen KM, Piedmonte MR: Influence of variations in projection geometry and lesion size on detection of computer-simulated crestal alveolar bone lesions by subtraction radiography. J Periodont Res 1991;26:48–51.
55 Hausmann E, Allen K, Carpio L, Christersson LA, Clerehugh V: Computerized methodology for detection of alveolar crestal bone loss from serial intraoral radiographs. J Periodontol 1992;63:657–662.
56 Albandar JM: Validity and reliability of alveolar bone level measurements made on dry skulls. J Clin Periodontol 1989;16:575–579.
57 Matsuda Y, Geurs NC, Reddy MS, Okano T, Jeffcoat MK: Relationship of bone loss to clinical measurements of defect depth. J Dent Res 1998;77(Sp. Iss):2896.
58 Jeffcoat MK, Reddy MS, Webber RL, Williams RC, Ruttimann UE: Extraoral control of geometry for digital subtraction radiography. J Periodont Res 1987;22:396–402.
59 Ruttimann UE, Webber RL, Schmidt E: A robust digital method for film contrast correction in subtraction radiography. J Periodont Res 1986;21:486–495.
60 Braegger U, Pasquali L: Color conversion of alveolar bone density changes in digital subtraction images. J Clin Periodont 1989;16:209–214.
61 Reddy MS, Bruch JM, Jeffcoat MK, Williams RC: Contrast enhancement as an aid to interpretation in digital subtraction radiography. Oral Surg Oral Med Oral Pathol 1991;71:763–769.
62 Jeffcoat MK, Reddy MS, Magnusson I, Johnson B, Meredith MP, Cavanaugh, PF Jr, Gerlach RW: Efficacy of quantitative digital subtraction radiography using radiographs exposed in a multicenter trial. J Periodont Res 1996;31:157–160.
63 Jeffcoat MK, Reddy MS: Digital subtraction radiography for longitudinal assessment of peri-implant bone change: Method and validation. Adv Dent Res 1993;7:196–201.

64 Braegger U, Pasquali L, Weber H, Kornman KS: Computer-assisted densitometric image analysis (CADIA) for the assessment of alveolar bone density changes in furcations. J Clin Periodontol 1989;16:46–52.
65 Webber RL, Tzukert A, Ruttimann U: The effects of beam hardening on digital subtraction radiography. J Periodont Res 1989;24:53–58.
66 Jeffcoat MK, Reddy MS, Jeffcoat RL: A morphologically aided technique for quantitative subtraction of dental radiographic images. IEEE/EMBS 1990;12:2068–2070.
67 Reddy MS, Wang I-C, Jeffcoat M, Jeffcoat RL: Progression of bone and attachment loss. Are they related? J Dent Res 1998;77:391.
68 Jeffcoat M: Radiographic methods for the detection of progressive alveolar bone loss. J Periodontol 1992;63(suppl):367–372.
69 Hausmann E, Allen K, Norderyd J, Ren W, Shibly O, Machtei E: Studies of the relationship between alveolar bone height and probing attachment level. J Clin Periodontol 1994;21:128–132.
70 Papapanou PN, Wernstron JL: Radiographic and clinical assessments of destructive periodontal disease. J Clin Periodontol 1989;16:609–612.

Dr. Marjorie Jeffcoat, University of Alabama School of Dentistry, 1919 7th Avenue South, SDB 412, Birmingham, AL 35294–0007 (USA)
Tel. +1 205 934 4506, Fax +1 205 934 7901, E-Mail jeffcoat@uab.edu

Faller RV (ed): Assessment of Oral Health.
Monogr Oral Sci. Basel, Karger, 2000, vol 17, pp 73–129

Analysis of the Morphology of Oral Structures from 3-D Co-Ordinate Data

V. Jovanovski[a], *E. Lynch*[b]

[a] Department of Adult Oral Health, St. Bartholomew's and the Royal London School of Medicine and Dentistry, London, and

[b] Restorative Dentistry and Gerodontology, School of Clinical Dentistry, The Queen's University of Belfast, UK

Abstract

A non-intrusive method is described which can be used to determine the forms of oral structures. It is based on the digitising of standard replicas with a co-ordinate-measuring machine. Supporting software permits a mathematical model of the surface to be reconstructed and visualised from captured three-dimensional co-ordinates. A series of surface data sets can be superposed into a common reference frame without the use of extrinsic markers, allowing changes in the shapes of oral structures to be quantified accurately over an extended period of time. The system has found numerous applications.

Introduction

There is a clinical need for objective quantification of the shapes of three-dimensional oral structures such as the morphology of teeth, the position and contour of the gingivae, the surface characteristics of fillings and their adaptation to the teeth in which they are placed. This need is particularly evident in the field of conservative dentistry which is concerned with all aspects of the conservation and restoration of teeth as well as the whole care of the patient. Additionally, such care requires assessment not only of shape, but also of changes in shape due to, for example, the wear of teeth and restorations, plaque accumulation, gingival recession or gingival inflammation.

Much of this assessment has previously been subjective and reliant on the clinician's experience. Examples are the USPHS criteria for evaluating occlusal restorations [1] by which several aspects of a restoration are classified as ideal, acceptable or unacceptable based on the observations of two or more evaluators, or the Leinfelder method [2] in which an experimental cast is compared visually to standard casts calibrated for wear in steps of 100 μm.

Subjective methods are insensitive to small changes and produce few, if any, quantitative results. Consequently, numerous techiques for obtaining objective measurements have been developed. Sometimes the features of interest can be presented in a planar (two-dimensional) form, for instance by producing sectioned silicone replicas which permit lengths and angles to be measured from photographs magnified by a known factor [3]. However, the most useful and widely applicable techniques are those which provide numerical data in the form of three-dimensional co-ordinates. Such techniques include stereophotogrammetry [4, 5], reflex microscopy [6–8], laser interferometry [9, 10], scanning electron microscopy [11–14], microtomography [15–17], conforcal microscopy [18], infra-red cameras [19] and mechanical digitisers [20]. A review can be found in Chadwick [21] and a table of methods and accuracies in Bayne et al. [22].

From the point of view of conservative dentistry, the techniques of greatest interest are those which can provide three-dimensional co-ordinate data acquired from an entire tooth surface with sufficient density and accuracy to permit the construction of a computer model. Additionally, the speed of data acquisition must be sufficient to permit practical application in clinical research studies involving large numbers of subjects.

Each of the techniques listed above is well suited for its particular area of application, but fails to meet these requirements in one or more aspects. A satisfactory solution has been provided by a category of measurement apparatus known as 'co-ordinate measuring machines' (CMMs), many of which were developed in the 1980s for industrial quality control of manufactured parts. Most CMMs consist of a horizontal platform upon which the object to be measured (a tooth replica, for instance) is placed and 3-D co-ordinates are acquired from it by an active data acquisition component in the form of a mechanical stylus or optical probe.

A number of systems based on CMMs or devices of equivalent functionality have been employed in dental research [23–30]. Their application generally involves three distinct stages of work. Firstly, a replica or model of the study surface is produced. Depending on the specific system used, there may be a requirement that the material be non-elastic, electrically conductive or of a particular colour and reflectivity. Secondly, co-ordinate data are acquired from the model surface. Finally, the data are analysed to produce quantitative results.

The published reports vary in the emphasis and amount of detail given relating to the methodology, but it is evident that the analysis of acquired co-ordinate data has frequently been problematic due to the unavailability of software which would be specifically tailored to the needs of dental research. The use of software intended for other application areas can render the process impracticably laborious. Where specialised software has been written, little is reported about the mathematical methods employed. Mitchell and Chadwick [31] write that 'although clinical results derived from such techniques are reported within the dental literature, none of the dental papers to date has described fully the underlying theory'.

With this in mind we present a detailed account of the methodology, supporting software and clinical application of the system for dental co-ordinate metrology developed at St. Bartholomew's and the Royal London School of Medicine and Dentistry [32]. Emphasis is given to description of the supporting mathematical models and the software which permits researchers to perform their own analyses by providing: (1) visualisation of surfaces with realistic rendering to enable the identification of anatomical features of interest; (2) construction of cross-sections and measurement of lengths and angles on such cross-sections; (3) quantification of changes in morphology by comparison of sequential replicas, particularly depth and volume changes on hard tissue and gingivae, and (4) output of results in graphical and numerical formats.

Particular attention is paid to the 'superposition' (or 'registration') of data sets obtained from a sequence of replicas of the same oral structure taken at different times. Such data sets do not generally lie in the same frame of reference and their comparison requires the application of co-ordinate transformations (rotations and translations) by which corresponding anatomical features are brought into coincidence.

The material is presented here in the following sequence, which reflects the progression from clinical replication to numerical results:

Replication of the study surface

↓

Co-ordinate data acquisition

↓

Construction of a computer model of the study surface

↓

Superposition of sequential data into a common reference frame

↓

Measurement

Replication of the Study Surface

Materials and Methods

The physical characteristics and mode of operation of CMMs preclude their use directly in the mouth. However, the provision of dental care invariably involves the replication of oral structures at some stage and dentistry has developed materials for the accurate and safe replication of oral structures, together with clinical expertise to use them effectively [33, 34]. Silicone impression materials are ideal for the purpose in hand, having been widely researched to determine their safety for use in the mouth, their elasticity, their ability to replicate very fine detail and their dimensional stability [35, 36].

The replicas in our studies were produced by a procedure similar to the standard routine followed in patient care but appropriately modified to address the special considerations that arise from the intended purpose of measuring changes in surface morphology. In studies involving sequential replicas of the same oral structure over a period of time it was desirable that the co-ordinate data capture be performed with all replicas having approximately the same orientation. In order to recreate not only the surface of interest but also its orientation, a special impression tube was designed which could be repositioned within the mouth in the same orientation each time.

An aspect of a tooth was selected as appropriate for the study to be undertaken, usually the buccal or occlusal surface of a tooth, and a plaster model was constructed from an alginate impression (fig. 1). A 9-mm length of accurately machined square section, rigid brass tubing of 12- or 16-mm nominal internal width was selected according to the size of the area to be studied. The surface of the model was lubricated and the impression tubing positioned on the plaster model over the surface to be replicated, so that its long axis was approximately normal to that surface (fig. 2). Its periphery was modified as necessary using a stone or a file so as to approximate the surface reasonably well. A polymethyl methacrylate resin was applied to the outside of the tubing to ensure that there were no gaps between the surface of the tooth and the tubing and to facilitate the correct locating of the tube in the mouth itself on one or many occasions.

On a subsequent patient visit, the quadrant containing the study surface was isolated and the tooth was gently dried with air. The tube was then located in its position in the mouth, held firmly in place and a polyvinyl siloxane dental impression material (Kerr Extrude, SDS Kerr, Orange, Calif., USA) was then injected onto the tooth surface within the tube to fill the latter to excess (fig. 3).

When the impression material had polymerised, the tube containing the silicone impression was removed from the mouth. Approximately 3 min after

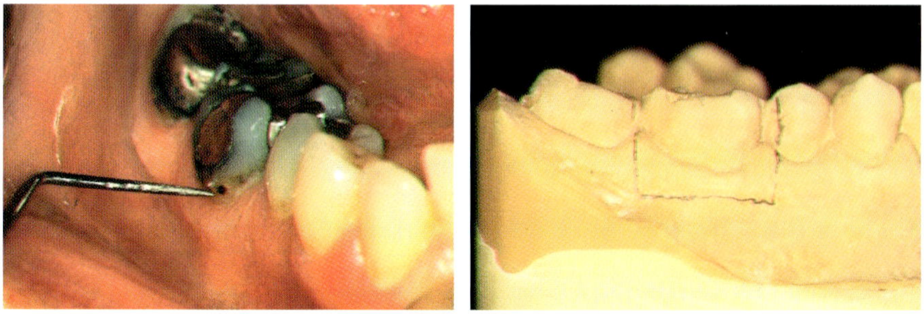

1

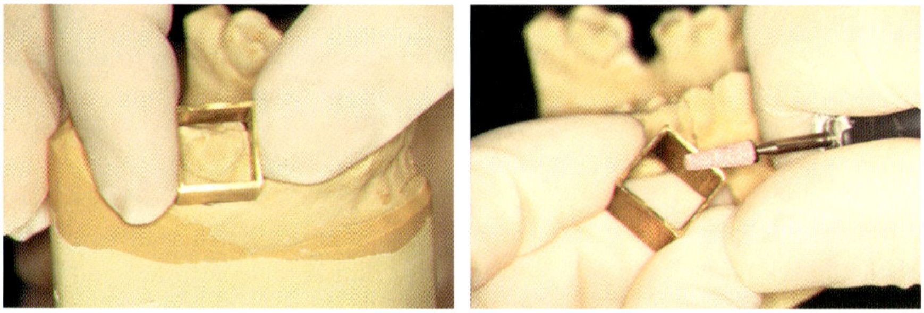

2

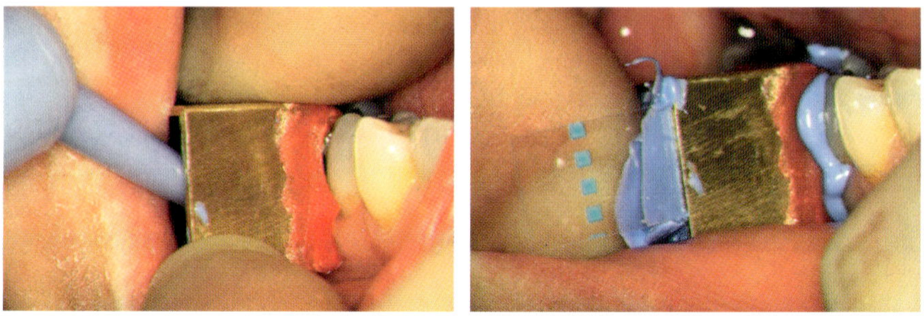

3

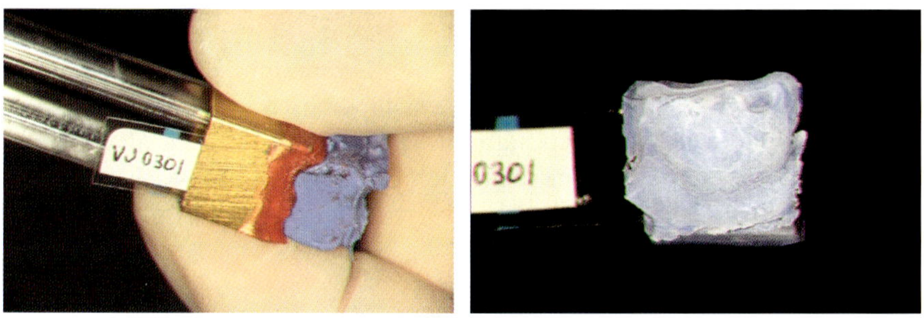

4

Fig. 1. The surface of interest identified in vivo and on the plaster model.
Fig. 2. Fabrication of the impression tube.
Fig. 3. Replication of the study surface.
Fig. 4. The completed replica.

Table 1. Repeatability of hard tissue replication

Study date	Number of pairs	RMS/point µm (mean ± SD)
1996	112	8.4 ± 2.1
1996	30	7.7 ± 1.8
1997	63	6.5 ± 2.5
1997	18	5.9 ± 1.4

this removal the base of the brass tube was trimmed flush with the edge of the tubing using a sharp blade and the block of silicone extruded from it. The tube was then available for further use on a subsequent occasion and the replica was ready for study (fig. 4).

Results

The physical properties of silicone-based impression materials have been researched extensively [36–40], showing their dimensional accuracy and long-term stability to be in the region of 0.1%. However, the replicas used in this work were not produced under the controlled conditions available in a laboratory, but in a clinical environment where they might be subjected to many additional influences. It was therefore considered necessary to perform our own evaluations of the practically achievable repeatability of sequential replicas of the same oral structure.

Sequences of repeat replicas were digitised and the data sets superposed into a common reference frame. Pairs of data sets were compared by evaluating the z co-ordinates of each of the data sets at 2,500 x–y locations distributed on a rectangular grid and recording the differences (which should ideally be zero). The measure of repeatability was defined as the root mean square (RMS) of the z differences, customarily termed the 'RMS/point' [30, 41]. Bearing in mind the procedures carried out to arrive at superposed mathematical models of the replica surfaces, the repeatability values obtained were all-inclusive, being influenced not only by the replication accuracy but also by the accuracy of the co-ordinate measurements, the superposition, as well as the instability of any soft tissue, e.g. the gingivae.

Hard Tissue

Table 1 shows the repeatability of replication of hard tissue over the course of several studies involving a total of 223 replica pairs taken at intervals ranging from 10 min to 6 months. Values which were found to differ significantly from these could invariably be attributed to the clinical procedure, for instance distortion due to failure of the replica material to polymerise fully.

Soft Tissue

Repeatability in the replication of gingivae was assessed on a series of 10 replicas taken in immediate succession. The pairwise RMS/point values were found to be between 29.0 and 64.5 (mean 41.8) μm. It is not currently clear what proportion of these differences in the sequential replicas of gingivae can be attributed to the physical distortion caused by the pressure applied during replication, and how much to changes in the gingival contour resulting from other factors including alterations in blood flow, desiccation or reactions to the chemicals within the impression material prior to its polymerisation. However, the repeatability of replication of the gingivae is sufficiently good to permit the investigation of changes in their contour caused by factors of interest in our studies, since such changes are generally considerably greater.

Plaque

The repeatability of replicas made in order to determine the location and thickness of plaque were comparable to those made on clean teeth. There was some concern that the plaque may be removed or disturbed by the replication process, but measurements of the repeat replicas indicated that any such effects, if they had occurred, would be too small to detect with our system. Furthermore, the clinical applications have confirmed that the accuracy is sufficient, for instance, to demonstrate the progressive accumulation of plaque over a period of 21 days and to detect statistically significant differences between the efficacy of two plaque-removal procedures.

Data Acquisition

CMM and Optical Probe

The central data acquisition equipment is a Merlin Mk II 750 Coordinate Measuring Machine (International Metrology Systems Ltd., Livingstone, UK) fitted with a Renishaw (Renshaw plc, Wotton-under Edge, UK) OP2 optical probe (fig. 5). The dimensions of the machine permit accommodation of a wide variety of differently sized objects, combining a large measuring volume (500 × 750 × 500 mm) with high accuracy throughout that volume. The worktable consists of a block of solid granite whose mass reduces the effects of environmental vibration. The position of the probe in each axis is determined to a resolution of 0.5 μm by a photocell which detects patterns on a stainless steel/glass grating. The accuracy of the position in each axis is 4.0 μm + L/275000 where L is the distance (in metres) travelled from an initial starting point. Control is provided by an IBM-PC compatible

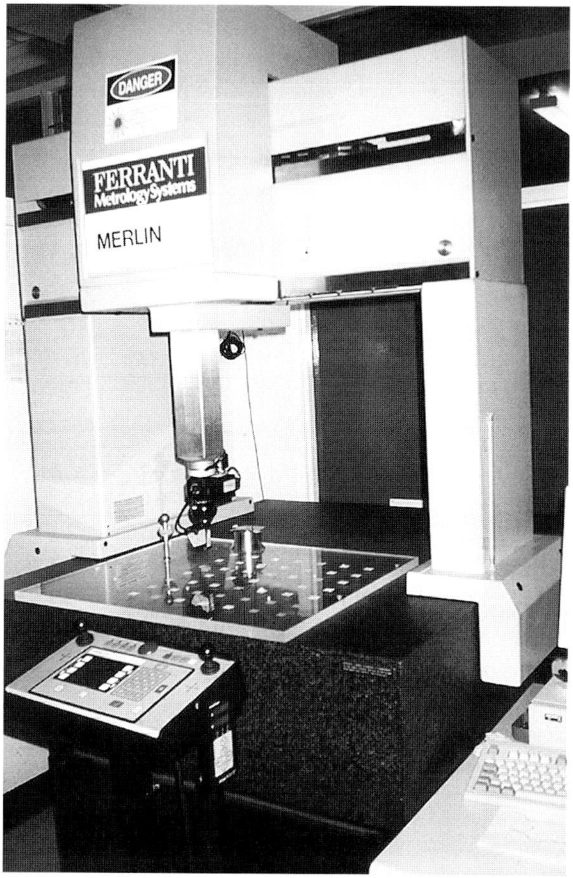

Fig. 5. The CMM and OP2 probe.

computer interfaced to the electronic desk unit which integrates the functions of the CMM and probe.

The Renishaw OP2 optical probe operates on the principle of 'optical triangulation' (fig. 6). A laser diode generates infrared laser radiation with a wavelength of 830 nm which is focused onto the surface, producing a spot 25 μm in diameter. The light scattered from the surface is detected by a position-sensitive device from which the surface height is computed. Each probe is individually calibrated and the calibration data stored in the controller firmware. The vertical measurement range of the probe is ±2 mm but this is effectively extended by the vertical motion of the probe column. Further flexibility in orienting the probe is provided by a multidirectional mounting which permits rotation of the probe around two axes. The maximum measure-

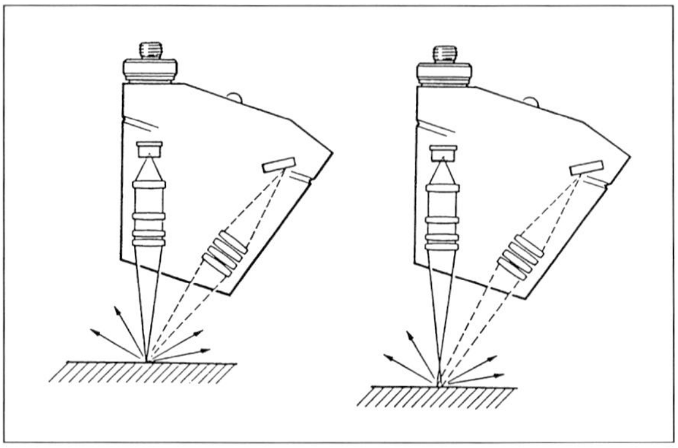

Fig. 6. Principle of operation of the OP2 probe. Copyright © 1988 Renishaw plc. Reproduced with permission.

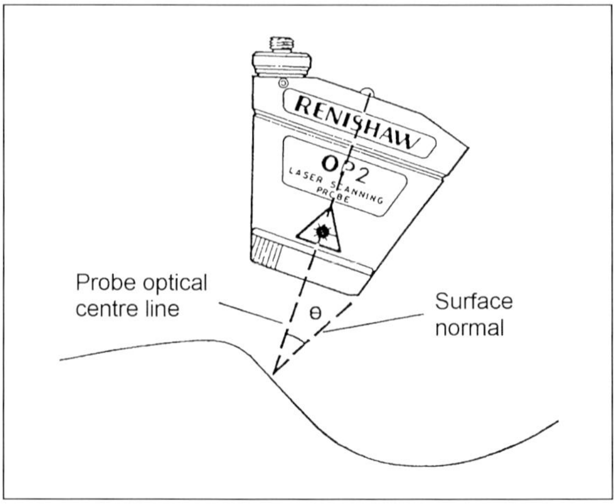

Fig. 7. The angle between the optical centre line and the surface normal. Copyright © 1988 Renishaw plc. Reproduced with permission.

ment frequency is 50 readings/s but in the integrated Merlin/OP2 configuration the optimal speed was determined to be 10 readings/s.

Two primary characteristics of a measurement device are its 'repeatability' (variations between repeated measurements) and 'accuracy' (how close the measurement is to the true value). The OP2 probe has a quoted repeatability of 2 μm. Its accuracy, however, depends on several factors, foremost of which is the angle between the probe's optical centre line and the surface normal (fig. 7), termed the 'gradient'. As the gradient increases, the intensity of the scattered light which reaches the detector decreases and the focused spot becomes elongated to an ellipse, which reduces the detection reliability. An optimal arrangement is achieved when the surface normal coincides either with the optical axis of the laser diode or with that of the detector and in such cases its accuracy is 5 μm.

A replica is digitised by programming the probe to move across the surface tracing a pattern of parallel 'scan lines'. The data point spacing (or 'scanning pitch') is most commonly selected to be 100 μm, with dimensions of a typical region of interest being 10 × 10 mm. Such a region requires around 25 min of processing time. The worktable can accommodate up to 36 replicas, placed on a 6 × 6 grid of squares, which can be processed sequentially without operator intervention. On completion of a batch of replicas the data sets are transferred to shared storage on a Novell NetWare (Novell Inc., Utah, USA) server where they can be accessed by all authorised users.

Repeatability and Accuracy

Familiarity with the capabilities and, equally importantly, the limitations of a measurement system allows it to be used efficiently while avoiding any temptation to extract meaningful information from unreliable data. The repeatability and accuracy are a complex combination of many factors and although it is convenient to summarise them in terms of single values, such summaries are not always realistic indicators of performance.

A series of experiments to establish the repeatability and accuracy of measurements in practice were carried out under standard operating conditions and on surfaces which were representative of those encountered in the clinical applications.

Repeatability was assessed by performing multiple measurements of a single replica. Since the OP2 probe is sensitive to the surface gradient, a labial surface which contained both mild and severe gradients was chosen (fig. 8).The replica was digitised four times. Within each region of interest (A–D), the *z* co-ordinates were evaluated at 2,500 locations and the standard deviation was computed for each location. Repeatability for each region was defined as the average of the 2,500 standard deviations. The results are given in table 2. As expected, measurements on steeper gradients were less repeatable, except in the case of region D which was not located on the smooth hard tissue.

The accuracy was determined by measuring objects of known shape and dimensions and also the replicas of those objects made from standard impression material. On a sphere of known diameter, the acquisition errors manifested themselves as progressive systematic deviations from the true values in accordance with the graph in figure 9, plus an additional random component which

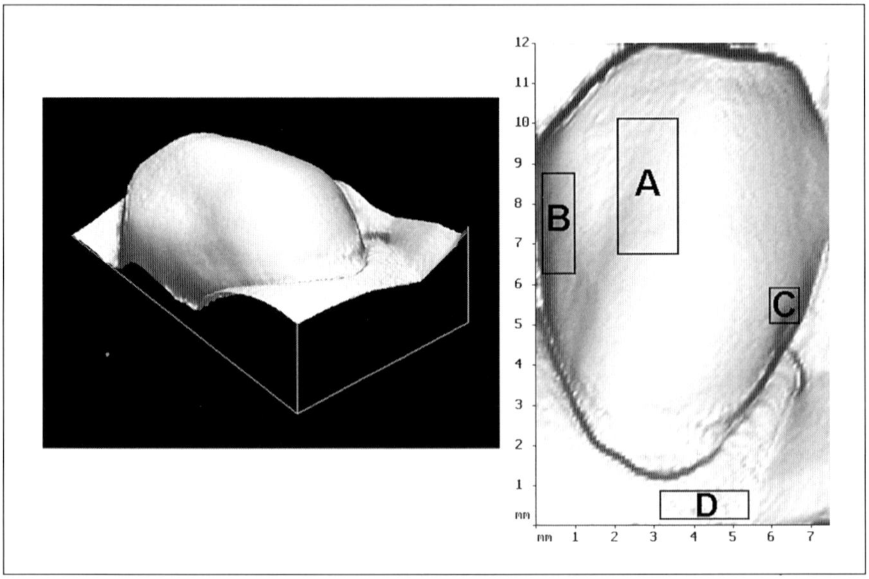

Fig. 8. Regions with different gradients.

Table 2. Repeatability on different gradients

	Region			
	A	B	C	D
Gradient	20°	52°	70°	20°
Repeatability, µm	2.4	4.0	5.3	4.5

is of a similar magnitude to the errors on flat, optimally oriented surfaces [42, 43]. The result of measuring a smooth surface was, therefore, again a smooth surface, although slightly distorted in regions with steep gradients. This had the desirable consequence of preserving reproducibility. Thus, when comparing sequential replicas of a single tooth, the difference between the two replicas could be determined to a greater accuracy (generally 5 µm) than could their true shapes.

It was also found that the probe's accuracy was not omnidirectional with respect to rotation around the optical centre line and that optimal results could be achieved if the probe travelled in a direction which was normal to the plane defined by the laser beam and the optical centre line [44]. The

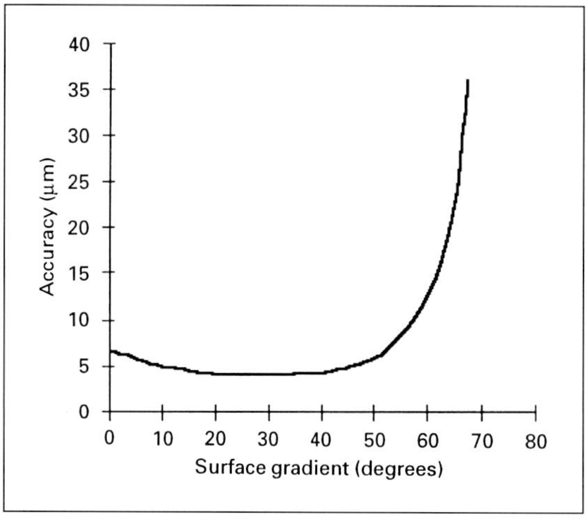

Fig. 9. OP2 probe accuracy vs. gradient.

standard procedure for digitising replicas was modified to take this aspect into account.

If a surface with a variable gradient is to be digitised without continually reorienting the probe, the best compromise is to orient the probe in such a way that the optical centre line is normal to the 'mean best fit plane' through the surface. Some surfaces can be processed using two or more probe orientations, but doing so requires additional operator effort and is not used routinely. In most applications involving single surfaces of teeth, the region of interest does not extend over too large a range of gradients and the replica can be positioned on the worktable in such a way that it is presented to the probe in a favourable orientation.

Although the error in z co-ordinates acquired on steep gradients may be relatively large (assuming that the probe is oriented so that its optical centre line coincides with the z axis), the errors of computed 'distances' are smaller when the dimension of interest is in a direction normal to the surface, for instance when measuring the loss of hard tooth tissue. If Δz is the acquisition error for a point on a flat surface inclined at angle α to the horizontal, then the error of measured distances Δd is only affected by that component of the acquisition error which lies in the direction of the dimension of interest ($\Delta d = \Delta z \cos \alpha$). If a replica is digitised in two different orientations, the average probe-to-surface angle will also differ and the measurements at any particular location on the replica will have been made under different accuracy conditions. Similar considerations apply when digitising two sequential replicas of the same oral structure. For purposes of quantifying morphological change, the two data sets can be brought into a common reference frame but doing so does not compensate for inconsistencies caused by acquisition errors which arise from the different probe-to-surface gradients. In practice this aspect proved not to be a problem for misorientations of up to 10°, an accuracy of positioning which is easily achieved by the operator.

The repeatability of measurements was found to be lower on regions whose contour changes rapidly over an interval comparable to the scanning pitch. This is not due to acquisition errors, since it occurs even with a theoretically perfect digitiser, but a consequence of the sparse spacing of the data points relative to the complexity of the surface contour. In relation to oral structures, this effect can occur to a small extent on gingivae, shown by the reduced repeatability for region D of figure 8. However, changes in gingival contour are evaluated over a sufficiently large region (>1 mm^2) for the height uncertainty to be greatly reduced by averaging. Thus, even with high-accuracy digitising systems, on certain types of surface features the sampling density is the primary determinant of accuracy and repeatability. The scanning pitch therefore needs to be appropriate to the surface morphology and the desired detail of information. In the literature, assessments of accuracy and repeatability of individual measurement systems are generally produced by measuring a flat surface, perhaps at several different inclinations. Such assessments should not be taken to mean that the values so provided are valid for 'real' tooth replicas, or that they are constant over the entire surface.

Reconstruction of Surfaces from Co-Ordinate Data

The data set obtained by digitising a replica consists of individual 3-D points (fig. 10). For the purposes of visualisation and measurement such a representation is not the most convenient or practical. For instance, one method of computing the volume enclosed between two surfaces is based on evaluating the difference in their z co-ordinate for a given x and y. This approach is not possible if the two surfaces were digitised over different x–y grids. The co-ordinate data therefore need to be represented in a form appropriate to the intended analyses. Since the orientation and movement of the laser probe during scanning are such that only one z co-ordinate is sampled at each (x, y) location, the natural form of a continuous surface that models the acquired data is a single-valued function $z = f(x, y)$.

The aim of surface reconstruction is to find such a function $f(x, y)$ which passes through the measured points exactly (interpolation) or as closely as sensibly possible (approximation) and which models the underlying surface

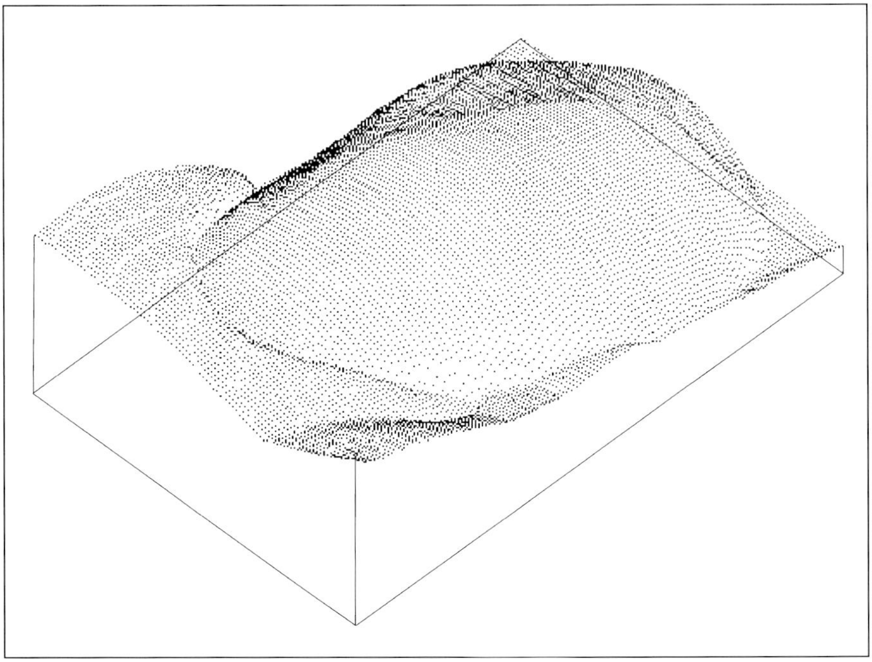

Fig. 10. A data set consisting of 11,432 points acquired from a labial tooth surface.

with sufficient accuracy in the regions between data points. The degree of success with which this can be done is dependent, amongst other things, on the accuracy of the measurements, their density (which should be sufficiently high to represent the smallest features of interest) and their (x, y) locations (more complex and time-consuming for non-uniform data). From a practical viewpoint, it is also desirable that the computation and subsequent evaluation of the function f be efficient and numerically stable.

Polynomial Splines

Consider the interpolation of a set of 2-D data points $A = \{(x_1, y_1), (x_2, y_2), ..., (x_n, y_n)\}$ obtained from measurements of a curve defined on an interval $[x_{min}, x_{max}]$ satisfying $x_{min} = x_1 < x_2 < \cdots < x_n = x_{max}$. We wish to find a function $y = f(x)$ defined on the same interval which passes through all the points of A.

The simplest solution is provided by the piecewise-linear function whose graph can be constructed by joining the successive points of A with line segments. This function is continuous but it is not smooth and therefore it cannot be expected to model curved lines accurately.

On the other hand, the n-th degree polynomial

$$a_0 + a_1 x + a_2 x^2 + \cdots + a_n x^n \tag{1}$$

whose coefficients a_i can be determined formally by solving the system of n linear equations obtained by substituting each (x_i, y_i) in turn into expression (1), passes through all the points of A, but its value between the data points may often exhibit spuriously large oscillations. Its behaviour is non-local in the sense that each coefficient is dependent on all the data points and even a small change in the location of any of the points will in general alter the appearance of the entire curve.

An intermediate scheme which is both sufficiently flexible and stable is one whereby a function f is constructed by defining different polynomials on each subinterval $[x_i, x_{i+1}]$. These polynomials can be of a low degree (often cubic) and conditions can be specified at the joins in such a way that the resulting curve has continuity not only of value, but also of its first and possibly higher-order derivatives. Functions constructed in this way are known as 'polynomial splines', a term which derives from the analogy with the draughtsman's tool of the same name [45].

The concept of polynomial splines can be extended to higher dimensions. Polynomial spline surfaces have found wide application in a diversity of areas including computer-aided design [46], reverse engineering [47, 48], terrain mapping [49, 50] and medicine [51]. On this basis they were considered appropriate for modelling oral structures whose shapes are almost arbitrarily complicated and which belong to the category of 'free-form' surfaces about which very few assumptions can be made. A concise introduction to the mathematical theory and practical implementation of polynomial splines can be found in Cox [52, 53], and with more detail in de Boor [54].

Polynomial Spline Curves

Polynomial spline curves can be expressed as linear combinations of basis functions known as 'B-splines'. In defining a spline on an interval $[x_{\min}, x_{\max}]$, we will consider that the interval is partitioned by N points $\lambda_1, \ldots, \lambda_N$ termed 'interior knots':

$$x_{\min} < \lambda_1 \le \lambda_2 \le \cdots \le \lambda_N < x_{\max}$$

and that additional points, termed 'exterior knots', are defined such that

$$\cdots \le \lambda_{-1} \le \lambda_0 \le x_{\min}, \quad x_{\max} \le \lambda_{N+1} \le \lambda_{N+2} \le \cdots$$

Most commonly, the exterior knots are selected such that $\lambda_j = x_{\min}$ if $j < 1$ and $\lambda_j = x_{\max}$ if $j > N$ and this will be assumed to apply here.

The interval $[x_{\min}, x_{\max}]$ is divided into $N+1$ disjoint subintervals $I_0, I_1, ..., I_N$ defined by

$$I_j = \begin{cases} [\lambda_j, \lambda_{j+1}) & j=0, 1, ..., N-1, \\ [\lambda_j, \lambda_{j+1}] & j=N. \end{cases}$$

A B-spline of order n, denoted by $N_{n,j}(x)$, is defined on the knots $\lambda_{j-n}, \lambda_{j-n+1}, ..., \lambda_j$ by the recurrence relation due to Cox [55] and de Boor [56]:

$$N_{n,j}(x) = \left(\frac{x-\lambda_{j-n}}{\lambda_{j-1}-\lambda_{j-n}}\right) N_{n-1,j-1}(x) + \left(\frac{\lambda_j - x}{\lambda_j - \lambda_{j-n+1}}\right) N_{n-1,j}(x) \qquad \text{if } n>1$$

and

$$N_{1,j}(x) = \begin{cases} 1 & \text{if } x \in I_{j-1}, \\ 0 & \text{otherwise.} \end{cases}$$

The B-spline $N_{n,j}(x)$ consists of polynomial 'pieces' of degree $n-1$ so, for instance, B-splines of order 4 are referred to as cubic B-splines. It is non-zero only on the interval $(\lambda_{j-n}, \lambda_j)$ and therefore if a function is represented as a linear combination of B-splines, altering any one of the coefficients will only alter the function locally, over the same interval.

A polynomial spline curve $s(x)$ of order n defined on a set of knots $\lambda_1, ..., \lambda_N$ is a linear combination of B-splines

$$s(x) = \sum_{j=1}^{q} c_j N_{n,j}(x)$$

where $q = N+n$ and $c_1, ..., c_q$ are 'B-spline coefficients'. Interpolation of a set of data points with a spline curve thus consists of selecting an appropriate grid and then determining the unknown B-spline coefficients from the conditions $s(x_i) = y_i$. Figure 11 shows a cubic spline curve

$$s(x) = \sum_{j=1}^{11} c_j N_{4,j}(x)$$

with $N=7$ interior knots. The B-spline $N_{4,6}(x)$ is shown in bold.

Polynomial Spline Surfaces

A polynomial spline surface is defined over a rectangular region $[x_{\min}, x_{\max}] \times [y_{\min}, y_{\max}]$. Taking each axis separately, denote by $M_{n_x,i}(x)$ the B-splines of order n_x for a set of N_x interior knots $\lambda_1, ..., \lambda_{N_x}$ on $[x_{\min}, x_{\max}]$ and by $N_{n_y,j}(y)$ the B-splines of order n_y for a set of N_y interior knots $\mu_1, ..., \mu_{N_y}$ on $[y_{\min}, y_{\max}]$. A polynomial spline surface $s(x, y)$ is defined as the sum of products of B-splines

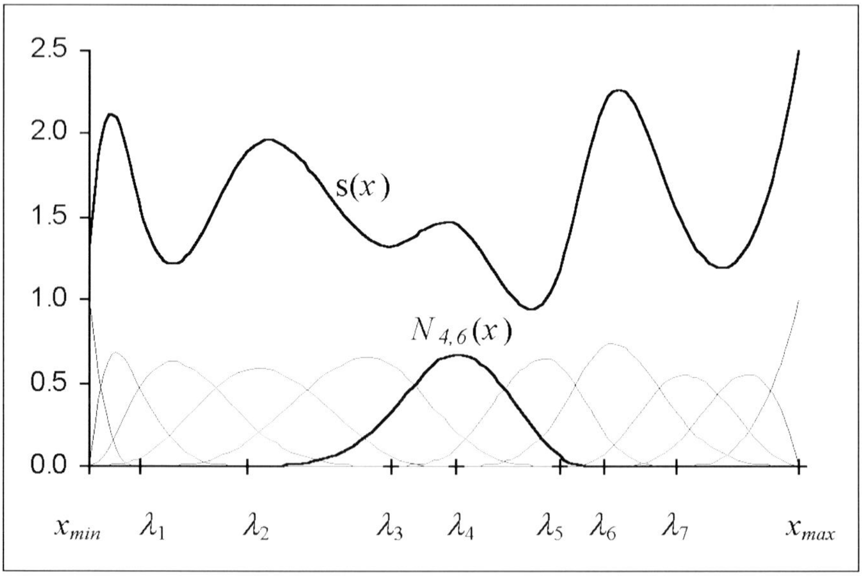

Fig. 11. A spline curve and the B-splines of which it is composed.

$$s(x) = \sum_{i=1}^{q_x} \sum_{j=1}^{q_y} c_{ij} M_{n_x,i}(x) N_{n_y,j}(y)$$

with coefficients $\{c_{ij} \mid i=1, ..., q_x, j=1, ..., q_y\}$ where $q_x = N_x + n_x$ and $q_y = N_y + n_y$. The process of constructing the interpolant of a set of data points (x_i, y_i, z_i) consists of finding the unknown coefficient matrix **C** by solving the system of linear equations resulting from the conditions $s(x_i, y_i) = z_i$. If the x–y locations of the data points lie on a rectangular $m_x \times m_y$ grid, then the coefficients **C** can be determined extremely rapidly and efficiently [53] by taking advantage of the separability of the system into the form $\mathbf{A}_x \mathbf{C} \mathbf{A}_y^{\mathrm{T}} = \mathbf{F}$ where $\mathbf{A}_x$ is the $m_x \times m_x$ matrix consisting of B-spline basis functions in x evaluated at the x gridlines, and $\mathbf{A}_y$ similarly for y.

Interpolation of CMM Data

As a consequence of the way in which a spline surface is defined as a sum of products of univariate B-splines, interpolation is straightforward only if the data points lie on a rectangular x–y grid. This is not the case with CMM data whose spacing is controlled by two parameters: the speed of motion of the probe column, and the frequency of readings of the OP2 probe. The two parameters are computed by the system software from a user-specified desired point spacing, but the actual achieved spacing is not guaranteed to be equal to this value, or to be regular. Additionally the laser beam need not be oriented vertically in which case the scan line is not straight but dependent on the surface contour. Whilst some CMMs are capable of producing data with constant spacing, this is not a great advantage since the rectangular distribution is generally lost if a data set is rotated in order to superpose it onto another. It was therefore necessary to consider methods appropriate for data points which do not lie on a rectangular grid.

Although any of the many existing methods for gridding generally scattered data could be applied, advantage can be taken of the fact that the data points are distributed on approximately straight lines [57–60]. The data set is regularised first in the direction of x, then in y by two series of successive univariate interpolations, resulting in a new data set, representative of the original, but which lies on a rectangular grid. This new data set is then interpolated with a bicubic spline surface as described above. Details are given by Jovanovski et al. [32]. The method of arriving at a surface representation by successive interpolations may appear to be a rather indirect way of constructing an approximant but there were practical reasons for this approach, foremost of which was the speed of execution. The software related to this project was required to perform with an acceptable speed on a wide variety of standard, modestly specified computers and this aim was achieved. A data set consisting of 10,000 points requires just 5.6 s of processing time on a Pentium 166 processor.

Accuracy of the Spline Interpolant

The spline interpolant of the gridded data points does not, in general, pass exactly through the original data points. The question therefore arises whether it is a satisfactory model. The data points are subject to measurement errors and there is therefore no great advantage in reproducing them exactly. It is suggested by Cox [53] that ‘an approximant should be sought that reproduces the data to the accuracy warranted by the data’. To determine if such an approximant was being attained, the residuals were evaluated on several types of replicas which were typical for the intended clinical applications and scanned with a pitch of 100 μm. It was apparent that the fit was worse in some regions than in others and that these regions were associated with detailed morphological features.

The root mean square residuals were found to be 0.09 μm on hard tissue, 1.95 μm on plaque and 1.06 μm on gingivae. These values were considered satisfactory. While it is possible to improve them further, for instance by applying the iterative method described by Anderson and Mason [59] and Anderson and Pink [61], it should be borne in mind that such improvements would be only in the numerical sense of fitting the surface model to the digitised

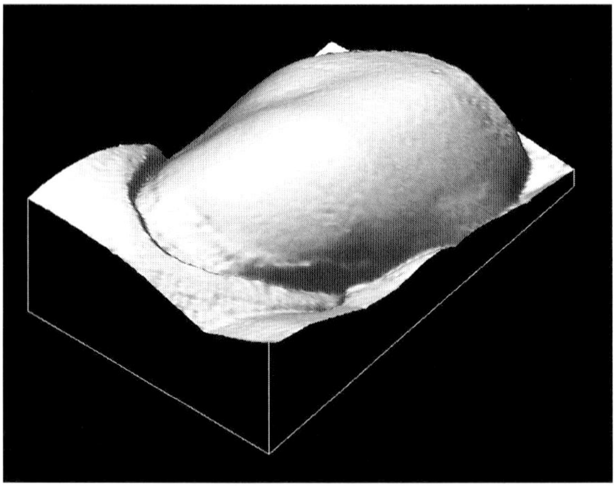

Fig. 12. The reconstructed labial tooth surface.

data and not necessarily produce a better representation of the underlying surface.

Visualisation and Measurement

When the surface has been represented as a continuous function $z = f(x, y)$, it can be manipulated in a variety of ways. Realistic rendering with Gouraud shading [62] permits the identification of anatomical features of interest and viewing of the surface in any desired orientation (fig. 12). Cross-sections may be defined by interactively marking a line segment which constitutes the x–y extent and measurements of lengths and angles may be made (fig. 13). The cross-sections need not necessarily be 'vertical' (i.e. parallel to the z axis), in which case the intersection between the plane and the surface is computed using contouring algorithms [63, 64].

Surface Representation in Other Dental Systems

Very little has been published about the surface representation methods used in other dental applications. Some systems permit digitising of a series of sequential replicas to be made on a common x–y grid by using external markers and mechanical repositioning. In studies of wear, it has been considered sufficient to evaluate the changes only at selected locations on the x–y grid and not on any intermediate points, which would require interpolation.

Cubic spline curves have been used in the development of the University of Minnesota system [65] to represent the surface as a series of parallel contours, and the intention of using bicubic splines for a 'full' surface representa-

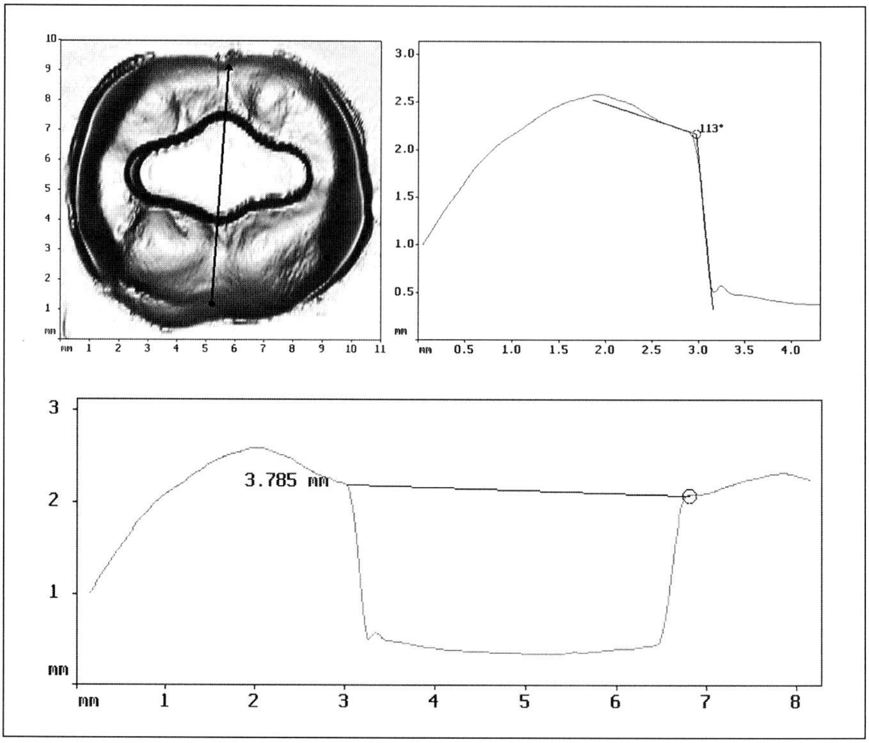

Fig. 13. Cross-sections, angles and lengths.

tion at a later stage was stated. In other systems, co-ordinate data sets are stored simply as an array of z values on an x–y grid. When a z value is required for point (x_0, y_0) not on the grid, a local interpolation is performed by fitting a polynomial through neighbouring points and evaluating it at (x_0, y_0). Most commonly, this has been bilinear interpolation (fitting a plane through three neighbouring grid points). Such is the case with the University of Munich system [30]. Mitchell and Chadwick [31] implement bilinear interpolation in the FORTRAN software, but refer to the possibility of using higher-order polynomials in the gridding of scattered data.

Although simple to implement, bilinear interpolation produces a less accurate surface model than quadratic or cubic interpolation. Furthermore, local interpolation can be inefficient since it entails solving a system of equations whenever a z co-ordinate is required. The speed of such computations is not critical in the gridding of scattered data since it is only performed once for each data set, but if z co-ordinates are to be evaluated at many locations, for instance during measurement, visualisation or superposition of sequential data sets, the advantages of polynomial splines, whose coefficients are pre-computed, are evident.

Superposition of Sequential Data

Mathematical Background

Comparison of two sequential measurements of the same tooth replica can reveal any changes over time, such as those due to plaque formation, caries or restorations. For such a comparison to be possible, the two data sets must be in the same frame of reference in the sense that corresponding points (those which represent the same anatomical feature) should have the same numerical co-ordinates. However, the co-ordinate data from any two replicas will not generally lie in the same reference frame. The two major contributing factors are: (i) variations in orientation of the brass tube assembly when taking the replicas, and (ii) variations in the orientation of the replicas when placed on the worktable of the CMM. Attempting to reduce these variations by physically constraining the positioning of the brass tube assembly in the mouth and of the replicas on the measuring platform is impractical since it would still permit errors whose magnitude is considerably greater than the dimensions of the intended measurements. The corrections to the orientation can, instead, be made retrospectively by applying to the (x, y, z) co-ordinates of the digitised surfaces such transformations which correspond to the physical motion of rigid objects. This approach can deal with all the causes of disorientation simultaneously and with high potential accuracy.

The process of bringing two data sets into a common reference frame in this way is known as 'registration' (the term commonly used in medicine and computer vision) or 'superposition' (elsewhere). The registration problem occurs in a variety of application areas including automated inspection of manufactured components, 2-D and 3-D medical imaging (with data from sequential observations or multimodal imaging) and computer vision (to determine the 'pose' of an object and recognise it by fitting to models of known categories of objects).

A Generalised Method

Suppose that a single image is printed on two transparent sheets but not necessarily in an identical orientation (fig. 14). If a person was asked to bring the two images into superposition, their most likely course of action would be to keep one of them in a fixed position and move the other one by rotating and translating so as to either bring the corners into coincidence, or maximise

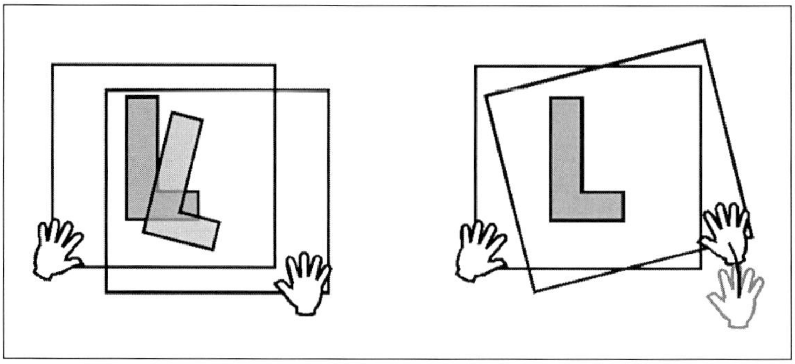

Fig. 14. Superposing two images 'by hand'.

the area of overlap. This procedure may be formulated mathematically as the following three-step 'generalised method': (1) express the position π of the second image relative to its initial position by a set of numerical parameters $u_1, u_2, ..., u_n$; (2) define a measure $E(\pi)$ of the positional disparity, and (3) determine the position of best fit by finding a vector of parameter values $\mathbf{u} = (u_1^*, u_2^*, ..., u_n^*)$ for which $E(u_1, u_2, ..., u_n)$ attains a minimum.

Unsurprisingly, these three steps form the essence of all registration methods encountered in practice. However, the specific choice of method for accomplishing each step depends on the nature of the problem as not all solutions will be equally appropriate to all situations. In the example of figure 14, two possible disparity functions were suggested: the first one expressed by the distances between the corresponding corners of the 'L' symbols, and the second one by the area of the non-overlapping regions. If the corners of the 'L' symbols were rounded, it would be difficult to identify corresponding points and the second function would be more appropriate despite its greater complexity.

Rigid Motion and its Parameterisation

Registration of two surfaces involves movement of one of the surfaces as a rigid body. In order to arrive at a parametric representation of the position of the surface relative to its initial position it is necessary to consider the class of those co-ordinate transformations which correspond to physical movement without deformation. Such transformations are termed 'rigid motion' [66, 67] and have the general form:

$$\tau(\mathbf{x}) = \mathbf{R}\mathbf{x} + \mathbf{v} \tag{2}$$

where $\mathbf{R}$ is a 'proper orthogonal' 3×3 matrix and $\mathbf{v}$ a fixed vector. A matrix $\mathbf{R}$ is proper orthogonal if $\mathbf{R}^T\mathbf{R} = \mathbf{I}$ (the identity matrix) and $|\mathbf{R}| = 1$. Such matrices are also termed 'rotations' since they corespond to the standard geometrical notions of physical rotation around the co-ordinate origin. Stated in geometrical terms, the characterisation 2 is: every rigid motion can be represented as a rotation around the co-ordinate origin, followed by a translation.

The class of rigid motions forms a group in relation to the composition of transformations: (1) the identity transformation $\tau(\mathbf{x})=\mathbf{x}$ is a rigid motion; (2) if $\tau(\mathbf{x})=\mathbf{Rx}+\mathbf{c}$ is a rigid motion then its inverse $\tau^{-1}(\mathbf{x})=\mathbf{R}^{\mathrm{T}}\mathbf{x}-\mathbf{R}^{\mathrm{T}}\mathbf{c}$ is also a rigid motion, and (3) if $\tau_1(\mathbf{x})=\mathbf{R}_1\mathbf{x}+\mathbf{c}_1$ and $\tau_2(\mathbf{x})=\mathbf{R}_2\mathbf{x}+\mathbf{c}_2$ are rigid motions, then their composition $\tau_2(\tau_1(\mathbf{x}))=\mathbf{R}_2\mathbf{R}_1\mathbf{x}+(\mathbf{R}_2\mathbf{c}_1+\mathbf{c}_2)$ is also a rigid motion.

When registration is performed, the 'disparity' function E (termed the 'objective function'), can ultimately be represented as a multivariate function of the elements of the matrix $\mathbf{R}$ and of the translation vector $\mathbf{v}$. However, the nine elements of the rotation matrix are not independent, but connected by the relations arising from the orthogonality of $\mathbf{R}$ and as such they cannot serve as the independent variables of E.

In general the elements of an $n\times n$ orthogonal matrix are functions of $n(n-1)/2$ variables [68]. In three-dimensional space, rotation matrices can be represented as a product of three rotations $\mathbf{R}=\mathbf{R}_3\,\mathbf{R}_2\,\mathbf{R}_1$ of the form

$$\mathbf{R}_1=\begin{bmatrix}1 & 0 & 0\\ 0 & c_1 & -s_1\\ 0 & s_1 & c_1\end{bmatrix}\quad \mathbf{R}_2=\begin{bmatrix}c_2 & 0 & s_2\\ 0 & 1 & 0\\ -s_2 & 0 & c_2\end{bmatrix}\quad \text{and}\quad \mathbf{R}_3=\begin{bmatrix}c_3 & -s_3 & 0\\ s_3 & c_3 & 0\\ 0 & 0 & 1\end{bmatrix}$$

where $c_i^2+s_i^2=1$ $(i=1, 2, 3)$. Geometrically, $\mathbf{R}_1$ is a rotation around the x axis by an angle φ_1 where $c_1=\cos\varphi_1$ and $s_1=\sin\varphi_1$. Similarly, $\mathbf{R}_2$ and $\mathbf{R}_3$ are rotations around the y and z axes, respectively. The explicit form of the product $\mathbf{R}_3\,\mathbf{R}_2\,\mathbf{R}_1$ is

$$\mathbf{R}=\begin{bmatrix}c_2c_3 & s_1s_2c_3-c_1s_3 & c_1s_2c_3-s_1s_3\\ c_2s_3 & s_1s_2s_3+c_1c_3 & c_1s_2s_3-s_1c_3\\ -s_2 & s_1c_2 & c_1c_2\end{bmatrix}.$$

Thus, a rotation matrix can be parameterised by three rotation angles [69]. On occasions where it is necessary to convert between matrix and parameter representations, the rotation angles can be found from the relationships:

$$\tan\varphi_1=\frac{r_{32}}{r_{33}}\quad \tan\varphi_2=\frac{-r_{31}}{\sqrt{r_{32}^2+r_{33}^2}}\quad \text{and}\quad \tan\varphi_3=\frac{r_{21}}{r_{11}}.$$

In summary, every rigid motion $\mathbf{Rx}+\mathbf{v}$ in three-dimensional space can be represented by a six-parameter vector

$$\mathbf{p}=(\varphi_1, \varphi_2, \varphi_3, v_1, v_2, v_3)$$

where φ_1, φ_2 and φ_3 are rotation angles and v_1, v_2 and v_3 are the components of the translation vector $\mathbf{v}$.

As outlined above, determining the optimum transformation requires finding the minimum of an objective function E which contains a rotation matrix $\mathbf{R}$ whose elements r_{ij} are functions of the rotation angles. Since the methods for minimising E generally require the evaluation of its partial derivatives with respect to the rotation angles, it is useful at this stage to define $\partial\mathbf{R}/\partial\alpha$, the 'partial derivative of a rotation matrix $\mathbf{R}$ with respect to the rotation angle' α, to be the matrix whose (i, j)-th element is the partial derivative of $r_{ij}(\varphi_1, \varphi_2, \varphi_3)$ with respect to α.

Specifically,

$$\frac{\partial\mathbf{R}}{\partial\varphi_1}=\begin{bmatrix} 0 & c_1s_2c_3+s_1s_3 & -s_1s_2c_3+c_1s_3 \\ 0 & c_1s_2s_3-s_1c_3 & -s_1s_2s_3-c_1c_3 \\ 0 & c_1c_2 & -s_1c_2 \end{bmatrix}$$

$$\frac{\partial\mathbf{R}}{\partial\varphi_2}=\begin{bmatrix} -s_2c_3 & s_1c_2c_3 & c_1c_2c_3 \\ -s_2s_3 & s_1c_2s_3 & c_1c_2s_3 \\ -c_2 & -s_1s_2 & -c_1s_2 \end{bmatrix}$$

and

$$\frac{\partial\mathbf{R}}{\partial\varphi_3}=\begin{bmatrix} -c_2s_3 & -s_1s_2s_3-c_1c_3 & -c_1s_2s_3+s_1c_3 \\ c_2c_3 & s_1s_2c_3-c_1s_3 & c_1s_2c_3+s_1s_3 \\ 0 & 0 & 0 \end{bmatrix}.$$

This notation permits expressions to be written compactly and in a form similar to that for single-valued functions of one variable.

Methods Based on Identification of Corresponding Points

The position and orientation of an object in three-dimensional space are determined uniquely by the locations of at least three non-collinear points on its surface. If pairs of corresponding points are identified on two surfaces, then the surfaces can be superposed by finding the rigid motion which brings the second set of points into 'best' correspondence with the first. In practice an exact match will usually not be possible, due to errors arising from measurement or from the process of identifying the corresponding points, so the notion of 'best' is defined in a least squares sense. The formal statement of the problem is: given two sets of points $A=\{\mathbf{a}_1, \mathbf{a}_2, ..., \mathbf{a}_m\}$ and $B=\{\mathbf{b}_1, \mathbf{b}_2, ..., \mathbf{b}_m\}$, find a rigid motion $\tau(\mathbf{x})=\mathbf{Rx}+\mathbf{v}$ which, when applied to B, minimises the sum of squares of distances

$$E(\mathbf{R}, \mathbf{v}) = \sum_{i=1}^{m} \| \mathbf{a}_i - \tau(\mathbf{b}_i) \|^2.$$

This problem has been considered by many researchers [69–73]. It can be shown that the optimal transformation has the form $\tau(\mathbf{x}) = \mathbf{R}(\mathbf{x} - \bar{\mathbf{b}}) + \bar{\mathbf{a}}$ where $\bar{\mathbf{a}}$ and $\bar{\mathbf{b}}$ are the centroids of A and B, respectively. Furthermore, if A and B are centred around the co-ordinate origin to obtain new data sets X and Y, then **R** is that rotation matrix which maximises the sum

$$\sum_{i=1}^{m} \mathbf{x}_i^{\mathrm{T}} \mathbf{R} \mathbf{y}_i .$$

The optimal rotation matrix can be found efficiently by singular value decomposition (SVD). The SVD of a real $m \times n$ $(m \geq n)$ matrix **A** is its representation in the form

$$\mathbf{A} = \mathbf{U}\mathbf{S}\mathbf{V}^{\mathrm{T}}, \tag{3}$$

where **U** is an $m \times n$ column-orthogonal matrix[1], **V** is $n \times n$ orthogonal and $\mathbf{S} = \mathrm{diag}(\sigma_1, ..., \sigma_n)$ where $\sigma_1 \geq \sigma_2 \geq \cdots \geq \sigma_n \geq 0$. Details of the SVD can be found in Golub and Van Loan [74] and algorithms for its computational implementation in Press et al. [75].

The matrix **R** which produces the optimal fit of the two sets of points X and Y is found as follows: (1) form the $m \times 3$ matrices **X** and **Y** whose rows are the co-ordinates of the points in X and Y, respectively; (2) form the product $\mathbf{C} = \mathbf{Y}^{\mathrm{T}}\mathbf{X}$; (3) compute the SVD $\mathbf{C} = \mathbf{U}\mathbf{S}\mathbf{V}^{\mathrm{T}}$, and (4) the solution is $\mathbf{R} = \mathbf{U}\mathbf{V}^{\mathrm{T}}$.

Because of its simplicity, registration by point correspondence has been applied extensively. In relation to anatomical surfaces (including teeth), there are two approaches to the identification of corresponding points: (a) external markers can be attached to the surface under investigation [8, 24, 76, 77] or made on the surface itself [28, 78], and (b) characteristic points (landmarks) can be identified on the surface anatomy retrospectively by presenting the acquired data on a computer visualisation system [79].

Both approaches were attempted in our laboratory.

External Markers

Three ball-bearing were permanently attached to a tooth throughout the course of the investigations. The acquisition of a large number of points on the surface of these ball-bearings permitted the co-ordinates of their centres to be computed and these centres served as the three required reference points. The co-ordinates of the centres could be identified to within 8 μm in x and y, but only to within 36 μm in z [80].

[1] If $\mathbf{u}_i$ and $\mathbf{u}_j$ are two columns of **U** then $\mathbf{u}_i^{\mathrm{T}} \mathbf{u}_j = 1$ if $i = j$ and 0 otherwise.

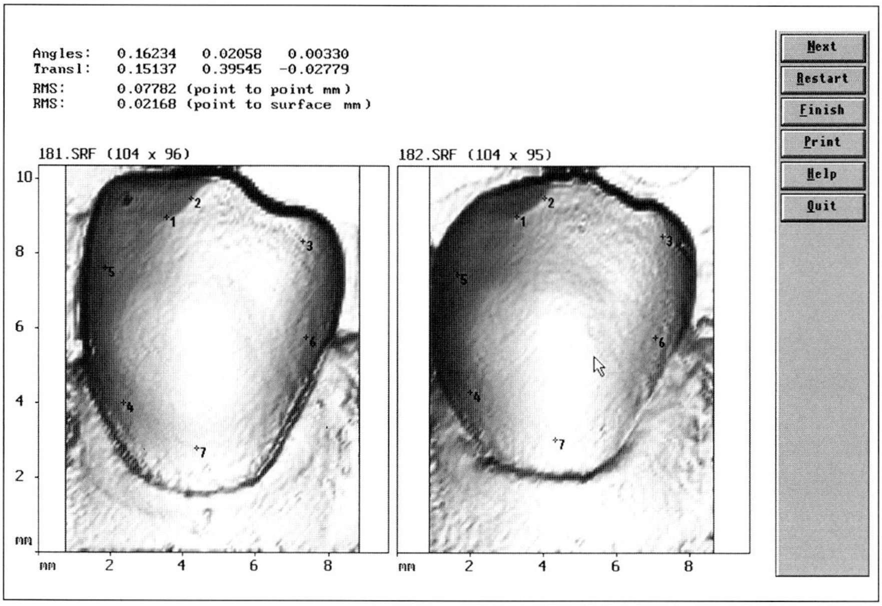

Fig. 15. Interactive identification of corresponding points.

This degree of accuracy was, however, insufficient. Such closely spaced reference points did not form a stable configuration for superposition since the errors in the computed transformation angles are inversely proportional (approximately) to the distances between the reference points. The clinical aspect was also problematic. External markers are uncomfortable for the subject and the oral environment may cause chemical changes to their surface. In a study of denture wear using a reflex microscope, Adams et al. [8] concluded that the markers 'should not be subject to any, even microscopic, changes of position, substance or definition during the monitoring period', since the registration accuracy could be seriously affected by any such changes.

Surface Landmarks

The software for surface reconstruction and visualisation developed for this project incorporates a facility to display a baseline and follow-up surface side-by-side and to mark points interactively on either of them (fig. 15). A point-to-point fit is performed and the computed transformation parameters are applied to the data points of the follow-up surface and re-interpolated to produce a bicubic spline surface superposed onto the first.

The accuracy ultimately attainable with this method was 10 μm [81], but only with great effort. The accurate identification of corresponding points was

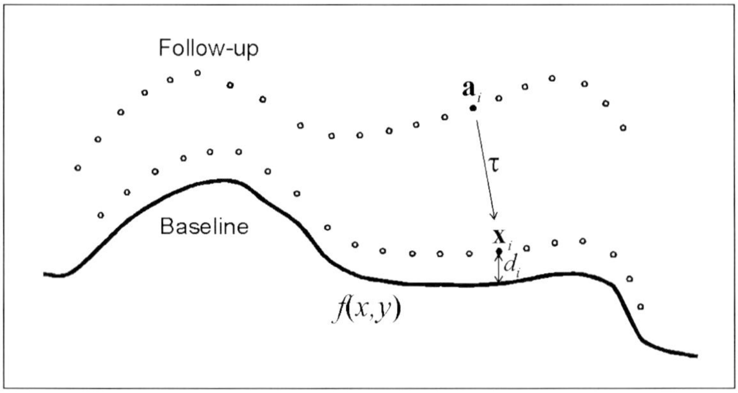

Fig. 16. Transforming a set of representative points.

limited by the resolution of the displayed image (30 μm/screen pixel) and by the relatively featureless morphology of some categories of surfaces, particularly anterior teeth. Partial compensation for both these sources of inaccuracy could be made by selecting a larger number of corresponding pairs, but the effect of one or two grossly mismatched pairs was serious [79]. However, this method is capable of quickly providing an initial approximation which can further be refined by other methods, described next.

Shape-Based Method

Methods based on the locations of landmarks, by their very nature, only use a small amount of the surface information. By utilising the additional information made available by the representation of the baseline surface as a continuous functions $f(x, y)$, it was possible to develop a method based on point-to-surface distances [82] which is robust and whose accuracy is operator-independent.

Suppose we are given a baseline surface $z=f(x, y)$ and a set of points $A=\{\mathbf{a}_1, \mathbf{a}_2, ..., \mathbf{a}_m\}$ selected from a nominally identical follow-up surface (fig. 16). We wish to fit the set of points A onto the baseline surface by applying a rigid motion $\tau(\mathbf{a})=\mathbf{Ra}+\mathbf{v}$. Denoting by $\mathbf{x}_i=(x_i, y_i, z_i)$ the images of the points in A under the transformation τ (i.e. $\mathbf{x}_i=\mathbf{Ra}_i+\mathbf{v}$), the aim is to find such a vector of parameters $\mathbf{p}=(\varphi_1, \varphi_2, \varphi_3, v_1, v_2, v_3)$ of the transformation τ that minimises some measure of the disparity E between the transformed points X and the surface f.

Let the function E be defined as the sum of squares of distances d_i between the transformed points $\mathbf{x}_i$ and the surface f. Leaving the particular choice of the distance function $d = d(x, y, z)$ unspecified for now, the following will hold true: (a) E is a function of the individual distances d_i: $E = E(d_i)$; (b) d_i is a function of the co-ordinates of the transformed i-th point: $d_i = d_i(x_i, y_i, z_i)$, and (c) x_i, y_i and z_i are functions of the transformation parameters: $\mathbf{x}_i = \mathbf{x}_i(\mathbf{p})$.

Therefore, if the set of points A is specified, then the value of E will depend only on the transformation parameters $\mathbf{p}$.

$$E(\mathbf{p}) = \sum_{i=1}^{m} d_i^2(\mathbf{p}) \tag{4}$$

Minimisation of the Objective Function

Expressions similar to equation 4 occur frequently when dealing with experimental data that contain normally distributed measurement errors, because a sum of squares is a maximum-likelihood estimator [75]. The problem of minimising such an expression is a 'least squares problem'.

Consider first the least squares problem where each function d_i is a *linear* function of its parameters $\mathbf{p} = (p_1, p_2, ..., p_n)$:

$$d_i(\mathbf{p}) = a_{i1} p_1 + \cdots + a_{ij} p_j + \cdots + a_{in} p_n - b_i \qquad (i = 1, ..., m).$$

The optimal vector $\mathbf{p}^*$ can be determined by the following method [74]: (1) form the matrix $\mathbf{A}$ whose (i, j)-th element is a_{ij} and the vector $\mathbf{b} = (b_1, b_2, ..., b_m)$, let $r = \text{rank}(\mathbf{A})$; (2) compute the SVD $\mathbf{A} = \mathbf{USV}^{\mathrm{T}}$, and (3) let $\mathbf{u}_1, ..., \mathbf{u}_n$ and $\mathbf{v}_1, ..., \mathbf{v}_n$ denote the columns of $\mathbf{U}$ and $\mathbf{V}$, respectively. Then, the optimal vector $\mathbf{p}^*$ is given by

$$\mathbf{p}^* = \sum_{i=1}^{r} \frac{\mathbf{u}_i^{\mathrm{T}} \mathbf{b}}{\sigma_i} \mathbf{v}_i .$$

The optimal vector $\mathbf{p}^*$ is also termed the solution of the overdetermined system of linear equations $\mathbf{Ap} = \mathbf{b}$ in the least squares sense because it has the property that $\| \mathbf{Ap}^* - \mathbf{b} \| \leq \| \mathbf{Ap} - \mathbf{b} \|$ for all vectors $\mathbf{p}$.

If the functions d_i are non-linear, then the minimisation of expression 4 presents a non-linear least squares problem, which may be solved by the Gauss-Newton method [83]. The iterations of the Gauss-Newton method are performed as follows.

GN1: Suppose that $\mathbf{p}_k$ is an approximation to the optimal solution $\mathbf{p}^*$. Let $\mathbf{J}$ denote the $m \times n$ matrix whose (i, j)-th element is the partial derivative

$$\frac{\partial d_i(p_1, ..., p_n)}{\partial p_j} .$$

GN2: use the SVD of $\mathbf{J}$, as outlined above, to find a vector $\mathbf{h}_k$ which is the solution of the system of linear equations $\mathbf{Jh}_k = -\mathbf{d}$ in the least squares sense, where $\mathbf{d} = (d_1, d_2, ..., d_m)$.

GN3: Set $\mathbf{p}_{k+1}=\mathbf{p}_k+\mathbf{h}_k$. The vector $\mathbf{p}_{k+1}$ is a better approximation to $\mathbf{p}^*$.
GN4: Repeat steps 1–3 until satisfactory accuracy has been attained.

The Gauss-Newton method can now be applied to the least squares problem presented by the fitting of a transformed set of sampled points to a surface. The vector of unknown parameters is $\mathbf{p}=(\varphi_1, \varphi_2, \varphi_3, v_1, v_2, v_3)$ and therefore the i-th equation of the system obtained in step GN2 will have the form:

$$\left[\frac{\partial d_i(\mathbf{p})}{\partial \varphi_1} \; \frac{\partial d_i(\mathbf{p})}{\partial \varphi_2} \; \frac{\partial d_i(\mathbf{p})}{\partial \varphi_3} \; \frac{\partial d_i(\mathbf{p})}{\partial v_1} \; \frac{\partial d_i(\mathbf{p})}{\partial v_2} \; \frac{\partial d_i(\mathbf{p})}{\partial v_3}\right]\mathbf{h}=-d_i(\mathbf{p}). \tag{5}$$

The partial derivatives of the distances d_i with respect to the transformation parameters $\mathbf{p}$ can be found by applying the chain rule (with indices omitted for notational convenience):

$$\frac{\partial d}{\partial \mathbf{p}}=\frac{\partial d}{\partial \mathbf{x}}\cdot\frac{\partial \mathbf{x}}{\partial \mathbf{p}}.$$

It is readily verified that

$$\frac{\partial d}{\partial \mathbf{x}}=\frac{\partial d}{\partial(x, y, z)}=\left[\frac{\partial d}{\partial x} \; \frac{\partial d}{\partial y} \; \frac{\partial d}{\partial z}\right]$$

and that

$$\frac{\partial \mathbf{x}}{\partial \mathbf{p}}=\left[\begin{array}{c|c|c|c|c|c} \frac{\partial \mathbf{R}}{\partial \varphi_1}\mathbf{a} & \frac{\partial \mathbf{R}}{\partial \varphi_2}\mathbf{a} & \frac{\partial \mathbf{R}}{\partial \varphi_3}\mathbf{a} & \begin{matrix}1\\0\\0\end{matrix} & \begin{matrix}0\\1\\0\end{matrix} & \begin{matrix}0\\0\\1\end{matrix} \end{array}\right].$$

The explicit form of equation (5) is therefore:

$$\left[\frac{\partial d_i}{\partial x} \; \frac{\partial d_i}{\partial y} \; \frac{\partial d_i}{\partial z}\right]\left[\begin{array}{c|c|c|c|c|c} \frac{\partial \mathbf{R}}{\partial \varphi_1}\mathbf{a}_i & \frac{\partial \mathbf{R}}{\partial \varphi_2}\mathbf{a}_i & \frac{\partial \mathbf{R}}{\partial \varphi_3}\mathbf{a}_i & \begin{matrix}1\\0\\0\end{matrix} & \begin{matrix}0\\1\\0\end{matrix} & \begin{matrix}0\\0\\1\end{matrix} \end{array}\right]\mathbf{h}=-d_i. \tag{6}$$

All that remains is to select an appropriate distance function $d(x, y, z)$. The 'true' distance from a point $\mathbf{x}=(x, y, z)$ to a surface $f(x, y)$ is the distance between the point $\mathbf{x}$ and that point on the surface f which is closest to $\mathbf{x}$, termed the 'foot point'. Finding the foot point is computationally expensive [84], but a first-order approximation can be used. If the surface f is considered to be represented by its tangent plane at the point $(x, y, f(x, y))$ which is the z-projection of $\mathbf{x}$ onto f, then the first-order approximation of the distance is given by:

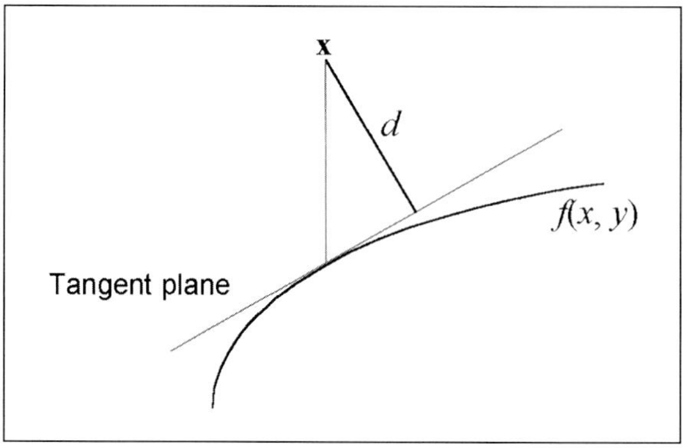

Fig. 17. A first-order approximation of the point-to-surface distance.

$$d = \frac{z - f(x, y)}{\sqrt{1 + f_x^2(x, y) + f_y^2(x, y)}}$$

where f_x and f_y denote the partial derivatives of f with respect to x and y (fig. 17).

Substituting this distance function into equation 6, the final explicit form of equation 5 in full is:

$$\mathbf{n}_i^{\mathrm{T}} \left[\begin{array}{c:c:c:c:c:c} \frac{\partial \mathbf{R}}{\partial \varphi_1}\mathbf{a}_i & \frac{\partial \mathbf{R}}{\partial \varphi_2}\mathbf{a}_i & \frac{\partial \mathbf{R}}{\partial \varphi_3}\mathbf{a}_i & \begin{matrix} 1 \\ 0 \\ 0 \end{matrix} & \begin{matrix} 0 \\ 1 \\ 0 \end{matrix} & \begin{matrix} 0 \\ 0 \\ 1 \end{matrix} \end{array} \right] \mathbf{h} = \frac{f(x_i, y_i) - z_i}{\sqrt{1 + f_x^2(x_i, y_i) + f_y^2(x_i, y_i)}} \qquad (7)$$

where $(x_i, y_i, z_i) = \mathbf{R}\mathbf{a}_i + \mathbf{v}$, and $\mathbf{n}_i$ is the unit normal of the baseline surface at $(x_i, y_i, f(x_i, y_i))$, i.e.

$$\mathbf{n}_i = \frac{1}{\sqrt{1 + f_x^2(x_i, y_i) + f_y^2(x_i, y_i)}} \left[-f_x(x_i, y_i) \;\; -f_y(x_i, y_i) \;\; 1 \right]^{\mathrm{T}}.$$

Superposition of Non-Identical Surfaces

In the preceding section it was assumed that the baseline and follow-up surfaces represent the same underlying shape, except for random measurement errors. However, the ultimate purpose of registration is to enable the measurement of changes in shape, and that fact implies that in practice the two surfaces will differ to some extent. The differences may be small (wear, for instance) or large (cavity preparation) but in most cases there exists a region which remains relatively stable throughout, or is subject to considerably smaller changes than those in the region of interest. The registration of

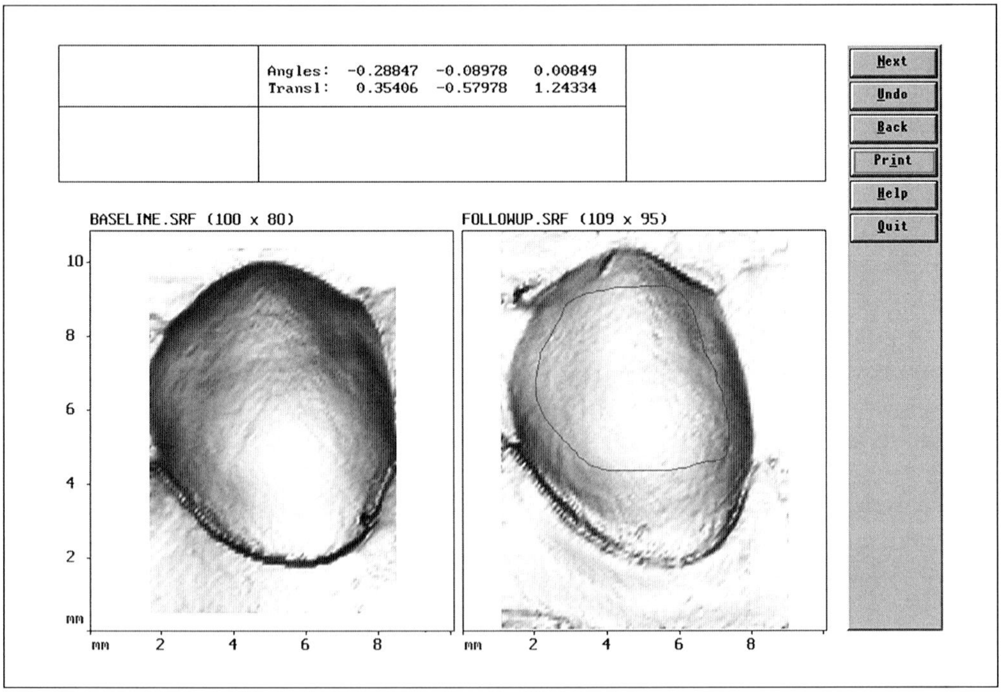

Fig. 18. The stable region outlined on the follow-up surface.

non-identical surfaces is achieved by restricting the selection of representative points to such stable regions. It is then possible to proceed as if the surfaces were identical.

Software Implementation

Registration is performed in three stages. First, an initial approximation of the transformation parameters is obtained by marking three or more pairs of corresponding points as in the landmark-based method, but with the difference that the points only need to be marked approximately because the method accuracy is not critically dependent on the choice of initial parameter values.

In the second stage, the operator marks the extent of the stable regions on the follow-up surface by outlining them with the mouse (fig. 18). The replicas in this example are from a study of the accumulation of plaque and changes in gingival contour. The crown was cleaned carefully using gauze, except for the region of interest in the proximity of the gingival margin.

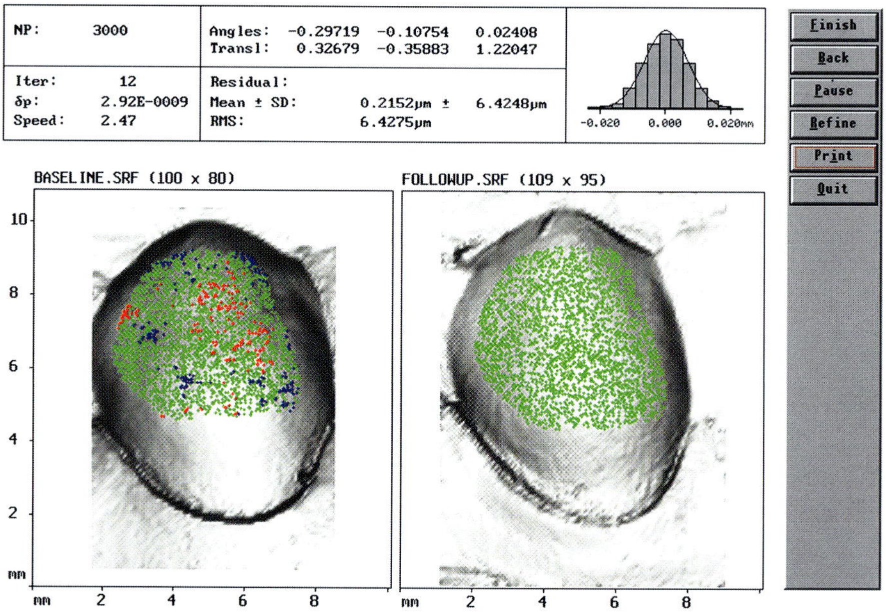

Fig. 19. The main processing phase.

On completion of the second stage, a set of 3,000 representative points which lie in the stable region of the follow-up surface is automatically generated by random uniform sampling (the number of representative points is chosen to be as high as possible, whilst maintaining an acceptable speed of operation). Following this, the main processing phase is initiated during which the representative points are fited to the baseline surface by the Gauss-Newton method. The display (fig. 19) is updated at each iteration to show: (1) the representative points, transformed by the parameter values obtained at the current iteration, overlaid onto the baseline surface: (2) a histogram of the distances (residuals) between the baseline surface and the transformed representative points of the follow-up surface; (3) statistics of the residuals (mean, standard deviation, RMS); (4) the values of the transformation parameters at the current iteration, and (5) the magnitude of their change $\delta \mathbf{p}$ from the previous iteration.

The primary indicator of a satisfactory fit is the RMS of the residuals (RMS/point). Additional verification is provided by the histogram. If the marked regions are indeed identical except for randomly distributed measurement errors, it is expected that the histogram should correspond closely to the overlaid Gaussian curve which has the same mean and standard deviation

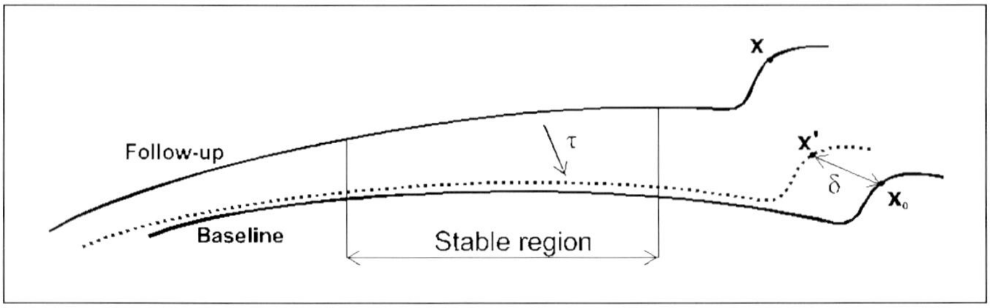

Fig. 20. Inaccurate registration, but low RMS.

as the residuals. Those transformed representative points which correspond to the worst 15% of residuals (outliers) are displayed in a different colour to the others (red for positive, blue for negative). The software incorporates a facility to exclude the outliers from further consideration and allows the iterative procedure to continue with the new 'refined' set of representative points. When the procedure has converged, the optimal transformation is applied to all the data points of the follow-up surface. From these transformed points a new, superposed follow-up surface is generated.

Results

The practical application of the shape-based method in a number of clinical studies involving many hundreds of replicas has shown that tooth surfaces can generally be superposed to within 6–9 μm RMS/point. The fit is not perfect because the registration is being performed on two surfaces which are not absolutely identical, as a consequence of the finite accuracy of replication and digitising. Furthermore, if a pair of surfaces are superposed repeatedly, the parameters of the computed optimal transformation will be subject to small variations, depending on the size and location of the marked stable regions, and also on the specific locations of the selected representative points. It was therefore of interest to quantify not only the overall goodness of fit, but also to determine which factors affect it, and to what extent.

Is some cases, the RMS/point deviation is not a complete indicator of the registration accuracy, a fact which has also been noted in other application areas [85, 86]. The example in figure 20 shows a situation where the stable region is an almost perfectly circular arc.

While the RMS/point value is low, the misregistration δ between corresponding anatomical features $\mathbf{x}_0$ and $\mathbf{x}'$ is high. From this it is clear that the evaluation of registration accuracy should be based on a measure capable of distinguishing between solutions which produce equal RMS/point values.

If τ^* is a known optimal registration and $\hat{\tau}$ is a solution obtained by some method, then the misregistration of a particular point $\mathbf{x}$ is the distance $\| \hat{\tau}^{-1}\tau^*(\mathbf{x}) - \mathbf{x} \|$, equal to the distance that a point $\mathbf{x}$ is displaced by the residual transformation $\tau_{err} = \hat{\tau}^{-1}\tau^*$. Clearly, the displacement is not constant for all points $\mathbf{x}$ due to the distance-dependent effects of rotation, but its average value can be estimated. Given a transformation τ whose parameters are $(\varphi_1, \varphi_2, \varphi_3, v_1, v_2, v_3)$ and a point $\mathbf{x}$, it can be shown that

$$\| \tau(\mathbf{x}) - \mathbf{x} \| \leq \| \mathbf{x} \| \sqrt{\varphi_1^2 + \varphi_2^2 + \varphi_3^2} + \sqrt{v_1^2 + v_2^2 + v_3^2} = \| \mathbf{x} \| \; \| \varphi \| + \| \mathbf{v} \|,$$

provided that the rotation angles are small, which is the case with τ_{err}.

The quantity $\| \mathbf{x} \| \; \| \varphi \| + \| \mathbf{v} \|$ is upper bound and scale-dependent. In our studies, with replica dimensions of approximately 10×10 mm centred around the co-ordinate origin, an appropriate 'mean' distance is 5 mm. We therefore define the mean displacement (MD) of a transformation τ as $\mathrm{MD}(\tau) = 5$ mm $\| \varphi \| + \| \mathbf{v} \|$. (Angles are dimensionless quantities, while vector norms are distances (lengths). The '5 mm' multiplier plays the role of $\| \mathbf{x} \|$ in the expression $\| \mathbf{x} \| \; \| \varphi \| + \| \mathbf{v} \|$. The MD is therefore also expressed in units of length.)

In this way, and assuming that the optimal transformation τ^* between two surfaces is known, the registration accuracy of a particular solution $\hat{\tau}$ can be defined as the MD of the residual transformation $\tau_{err} = \hat{\tau}^{-1}\tau^*$. In this context, the quantity $\mathrm{MD}(\hat{\tau}^{-1}\tau^*)$ serves as a measure of the 'distance' between the two transformations $\hat{\tau}$ and τ^*.

The repeatability of a sequence of solutions $(\tau_1, \tau_2, ..., \tau_n)$ is defined in an analogous way to the standard deviation of a random variable, as the root mean square of the 'distances' of each of the n solutions from their 'mean'. A transformation τ_{mean} is obtained by averaging the n vectors of transformation parameters, and the repeatability is defined as:

$$\text{Repeatability} = \mathrm{RMS}(\mathrm{MD}(\tau_k^{-1}\tau_{mean}), k = 1, ..., n).$$

A series of experiments to assess the accuracy and repeatability of registration were performed using data from actual digitised replicas of labial surfaces and also from surfaces generated synthetically. Each experiment was repeated 50 times with different initial transformation parameters which simulated the variations that would arise in practice from the landmark-based initial approximation phase.

Synthesised 'Typical' Case

Evaluation of registration accuracy requires that the exact solution (ground truth) be known, but this is not achievable with pairs of surfaces obtained by the standard procedure. Instead, a transformation τ was applied to a single data set P_1, obtained from a labial tooth surface, to create a new data set P_2. The two sets of points were interpolated to create two continuous surfaces S_1 and S_2. These two surfaces were 'digitised' synthetically by sampling two sets of data points D_1 and D_2 in such a way that their x–y distribution resembled that which would be obtained with the CMM. Random errors which modelled the characteristics of the OP2 probe were added to their z co-ordinates. Finally, the data sets D_1 and D_2 were interpolated to create a pair of surfaces related by the known transformation τ. When the two surfaces were superposed in the standard way, the accuracy, repeatability and RMS/point were 9.8, 8.1 and 6.4 μm, respectively.

Effects of the Distribution of Acquired Data Points

When replicas are digitised repeatedly, the x–y distribution of each set of data points is different and the spline interpolants of those data sets therefore also differ to a small extent. The accuracy, repeatability and RMS/point of data sets obtained synthetically from a single surface, but sampled at different x–y locations, were found to be 1.25, 1.26 and 1.24 μm, respectively.

Effects of the Locations of Representative Points

Repeated registration of two 'real' data sets was performed with different initial parameters, but with the same set of representative points each time. The repeatability was found to be near-perfect (10^{-4} μm). From this, two conclusions follow.

(1) Different representative points produce different solutions. This is expected, since the 'follow-up' structure represented by these points is different each time to an extent dependent on the accuracy of replication and measurement.

(2) The same solution was obtained each time, despite the different initial parameters. Therefore, no local minima of the objective function were encountered. It is generally found in other application areas that 3-D registration of free-form surfaces is sensitive to local minima, particularly with structures whose morphology is detailed, such as human brains. In such situations the global minimum can be sought either by repeating the superposition many times and rejecting 'outlier' solutions, or by parameter space searching. However, in this application the surfaces were smooth and the measurement errors low in relation to the data point spacing and therefore the solution was not sensitive to the choice of initial transformation parameters.

Effects of the Number of Representative Points

Since the information used in superposing the follow-up surface consists only of its representative points, it was expected that selecting a larger number of points would provide a better description and therefore a more stable and

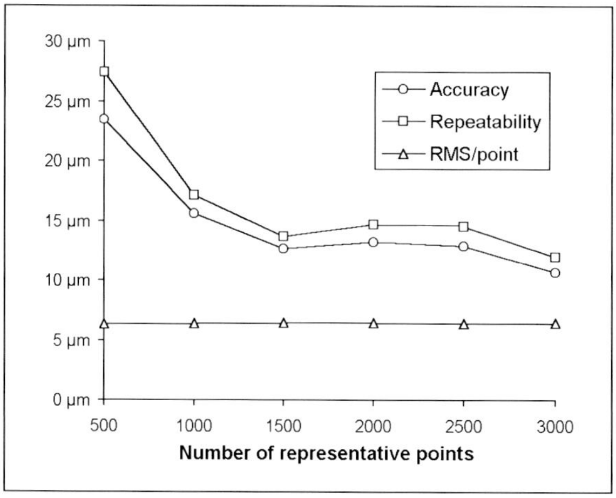

Fig. 21. Registration accuracy and repeatability vs. number of representative points.

accurate fit. Varying their number from 500 to 3,000 produced the results in figure 21. Better solutions were indeed obtained by selecting a greater number of points, but it was also apparent that an increase in their number above 1,500 yielded only slight improvements. These facts would not have been revealed by examining the RMS/point value alone, since it remained constant.

Effects of the Magnitude of Acquisition Errors

The sequence of operations employed to evaluate the 'typical' case were performed with different magnitudes of synthetic acquisition errors. The graph in figure 22 shows that a linear dependence exists between the acquisition errors and the RMS/point, but that the effect on accuracy and repeatability was proportionally greater. It is not yet clear why this should be so, but it indicates (as does the previous experiment) that the RMS/point value alone does not always provide all the information of interest.

Convergence Properties

The values of the six-dimensional vector **p** of transformation parameters at each iteration of the Gauss-Newton method form an iterative sequence $\mathbf{p}_1$, $\mathbf{p}_2$, ... which converges toward some optimal value $\mathbf{p}^*$ (within the bounds of the computing precision). The convergence properties of these sequences were of interest because this information might reveal deficiencies or indicate how the speed of operation could be improved.

A fundamental characteristic of convergent iterative sequences is the 'order of convergence', defined as the largest number r for which

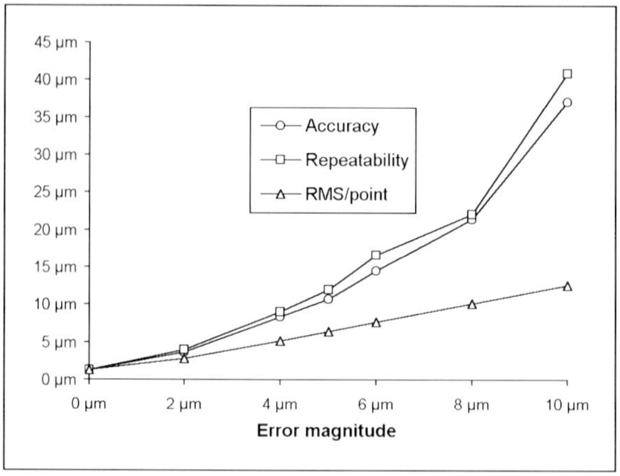

Fig. 22. Registration accuracy and repeatability vs. magnitude of acquisition errors.

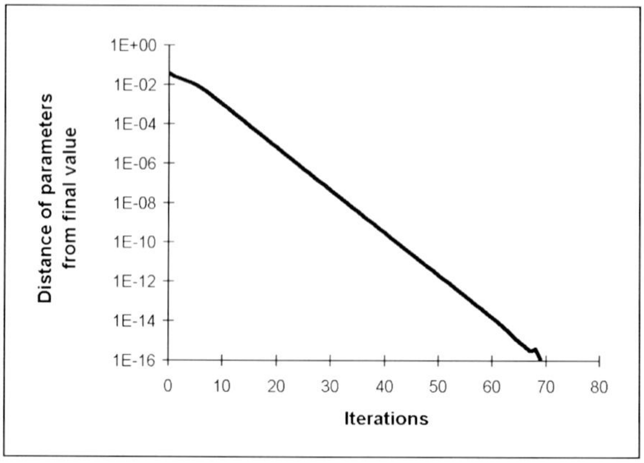

Fig. 23. The distances $\| \mathbf{p}_k - \mathbf{p}^* \|$.

$$0 \leq \lim_{k \to \infty} \frac{\| \mathbf{p}_{k+1} - \mathbf{p}^* \|}{\| \mathbf{p}_k - \mathbf{p}^* \|^r} \leq \infty.$$

The Gauss-Newton method is ultimately capable of achieving a quadratic rate of convergence, but only if the objective function tends to zero as $\mathbf{p}_k$ approaches $\mathbf{p}^*$. Otherwise its convergence is linear, and this was found to apply in the case of replica surfaces. The distances $\| \mathbf{p}_k - \mathbf{p}^* \|$ obtained during several runs of the registration procedure were recorded and plotted on a logarithmic scale against the iteration count. In each case, an almost exactly straight line was obtained (figure 23), showing that the ratio $\| \mathbf{p}_{k+1} - \mathbf{p}^* \| / \| \mathbf{p}_k - \mathbf{p}^* \|$ was almost constant.

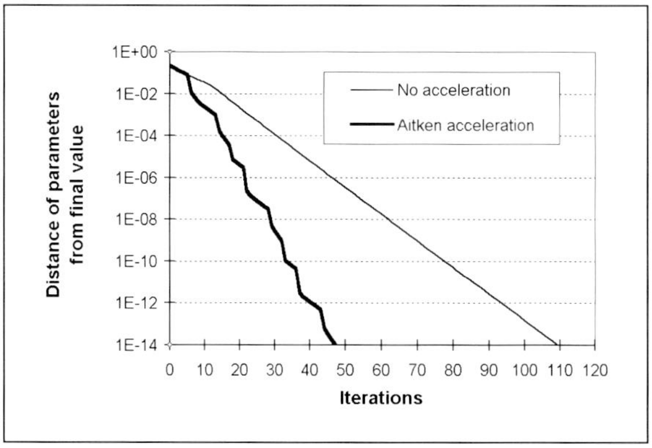

Fig. 24. Aitken acceleration of a slowly converging sequence.

The linear convergence permitted the application of a predictive technique known as Aitken acceleration to considerably reduce the number of required iterations. Consider a sequence $\{a_k\}$ which converges linearly towards a value a^* and in which each element is generated from the preceding one by some iterative procedure P. From the definition of the order of convergence it follows that for any three successive values a_{k-2}, a_{k-1} and a_k the following will hold true:

$$\frac{a_{k-1}-a^*}{a_{k-2}-a^*} \approx \frac{a_k-a^*}{a_{k-1}-a^*}. \tag{8}$$

The relationship 8 permits the approximate value of the unknown value a^* to be found as:

$$a^* \approx a_k - \frac{(a_k-a_{k-1})^2}{a_k-2a_{k-1}+a_{k-2}}. \tag{9}$$

The computed value of a^* is not exact, but if this value is used as the next element a_{k+1} in the sequence, instead of the value of a_{k+1} which would have been obtained by applying the procedure P, the convergence is greatly accelerated. Aitken acceleration has been implemented in the registration software and figure 24 shows the result of its application to a surface pair for which the convergence was particularly slow, resulting in an execution time of 30 s on a Pentium 166 processor.

Accuracy and Repeatability

The experimental results showed that the method error was negligible when applied to identical surfaces, and that the registration accuracy depends primarily on the accuracy of the acquired data. In the absence of a known ground truth, all registration methods are ultimately statistical [87], and while it is not easy to assess the accuracy of any particular solution, repeated registration of synthetically generated data sets, which closely model the real data, has provided estimates of what may be expected in practice.

An additional factor, not considered in the experiments, relates to the size, shape and location of the stable regions from which the representative points are selected. This is a complex issue which proved very difficult to quantify rigorously since the stable regions may be either single or multiple, with varying size and patterns of spacing. This question is closely related to that of ill-posed problems such as the example in figure 20, where the RMS/point remains constant or changes very slowly relative to the changes in the transformation parameters. It is well known that some categories of surfaces cannot be superposed uniquely. For example, a cone is invariant under rotation around its axis and therefore the superposition of two cones has one rotational degree of freedom. Similar considerations apply to spheres, cylinders, planes and other forms which are self-similar, i.e. invariant under some rigid motion. When such surfaces are superposed, the matrix $\mathbf{J}$ of the associated least squares system $\mathbf{Jh}=\mathbf{d}$ is singular and permits an infinity of solutions. Such surfaces did not occur in our investigations, since the measurement errors introduce sufficient imperfections to disrupt the geometrical regularity, but it was noted that selecting very flat or cylindrical representative regions caused slower convergence and worse repeatability. Despite the potential for labial tooth surfaces to be self-similar, there are extenuating circumstances. Measurements of changes due to plaque or wear are generally made in the z direction which represents the direction of maximum constraint and therefore they are not strongly affected by registration errors in the direction of maximum freedom. Given the fact that motion-invariance is an inherent property of the surface shape, it would be desirable to develop a method which would provide an *a priori* estimate of registration accuracy and stability. Recent work in other application areas has produced some promising results [88, 89].

Identification of Stable Regions and Removal of Outliers

The registration of non-identical surfaces is based on the assumption that stable regions exist and that they can be identified. The locations and extents of such regions differ depending on the type of change being studied and therefore some clinical knowledge of the problem is required, but there is always the possibility that the regions which have been marked as identical are, in fact, different. Possible causes are: (1) erroneous assumptions about the extent of the stable regions; (2) the presence of plaque or saliva on the tooth surface; (3) air bubbles on the replica surface, and (4) distortion of the replica caused by moving the impression tray at the critical stage while the impression material is setting.

The software provides facilities for the identification and rectification of such occurrences. If the differences between the marked regions are due only to measurement errors, then the RMS residual of the fitted points is expected to be in the range of 6–9 μm, the histogram of the residuals should exhibit a Gaussian distribution and the outlier points (both positive and negative) should be distributed uniformly.

If the outlier points are concentrated within a very small area, indicating a local fault, the operator can specify that they be automatically removed from the set of representative points and thereby excluded from further consideration. Larger regions of outlier concentration indicate more serious problems requiring further investigation which might lead either to the rejection of one or both of the replicas, or reconsideration of the possible locations of the stable regions.

Outlier removal has been used in other surface registration applications, including dental-related ones [30, 31] as a step towards automating the detection of stable regions, but there are difficulties with this approach. Namely, when the criteria for outlier detection are applied, the two surfaces are not yet correctly superposed, or there would be no need to take further action. The point-to-surface distances of the representative points will therefore differ from their final optimal values, permitting two types of classification errors to occur. Firstly, there might be failure to detect points which are not outliers according to the current relative attitude of the two surfaces, but would be if the surfaces were correctly superposed. Secondly, some 'good' points might be wrongly identified as outliers and rejected, thereby reducing the amount of available information. For these reasons, the registration software leaves the process of outlier removal under the control of the operator, to be used only where appropriate, such as in compensating for local imperfections.

Other Registration Methods

The development of surface registration methods has largely been motivated by the requirements of computer vision, industrial inspection and image-guided surgery. It can be seen from literature surveys [90, 91] that such methods essentially conform to the template of the 'generalised method', but that the specifics of each method depend on the properties of the acquired data. For instance, computer-aided tomography produces a 3-D data set whereby an object is represented as a large number of small cubes, each of which is assigned a discrete density value. Clearly, such data and the errors associated with its acquisition are of a very different nature to the tooth surface co-ordinate data and therefore require different processing methods.

Of methods that are applicable to co-ordinate data and surfaces reconstructed from it, the best known is probably the iterative closest point (ICP) method [92]. The ICP method is based on the fitting of two sets of corresponding points, as follows: (1) select a set of representative points on the follow-up surface; (2) for each follow-up point, find the point on the baseline surface which is closest to it; (3) fit the follow-up points to the baseline points, and (4) repeat steps 2–3 until convergence.

This method is popular because it is equally applicable to 2-D curves, '$2^1/_2$-D' (single-valued) surfaces and 3-D surfaces in general. It does not require the derivatives of the surface function to be known or estimated and permits straightforward implementation, the main requirement being a function which returns the closest point and a routine for least squares fitting of two sets of points.

The ICP method was implemented in our data analysis software as an alternative, but found to be inefficient for the following reasons: (1) finding the closest point is time-consuming [84], and (2) the presence of flat horizontal regions tends to 'anchor' the surface vertically which causes very slow convergence.

The method of Chen and Medioni [93] is a close counterpart of the method used in this work. This method, too, is based on minimising the distances from points to tangent planes, but whereas our plane passes through the control point $(x, y, f(x, y))$ (fig. 17), the control point in Chen and Medioni is chosen at the intersection of the baseline surface and a line through (x, y, z) which is normal to the transformed follow-up surface. The computation of this surface-to-line intersection incurs a considerable computational expense.

A point-to-surface method frequently cited in the medical literature is the method of Pelizzari et al. [94, 95] which has been used in brain imaging. The baseline surface is represented as a series of parallel contour lines and the follow-up surface as a set of points. The minimisation is performed by a parameter search method, which is reflected in the lengthy execution time, quoted as 'several minutes' for a set of 300 points on a VAX-11/750 computer.

In dental-related applications, Bangerter et al. [27] have used the simplex algorithm (also known as Nelder and Mead's polytope method) [96] for superposing tooth surfaces, but no further particulars are given. The University of

Minnesota system [97] also employs the simplex algorithm with a reported registration accuracy of 16.9 μm RMA/point on buccal surfaces [98]. The method accuracy of the latter is quoted as 3.5 μm [99].

The simplex algorithm is a parameter search method. As such, it does not require the derivatives of the objective function to be known or approximated, but its convergence is very slow. It was considered in the early stages of this work, but rejected after tests which showed that the superposition of two identical curves required over 100 iterations.

Dastane et al. [41] have performed a comparative study of three registration methods using commercially available software. The best achievable result in terms of RMS/point was 9.49 μm on surfaces defined by points on an 81×81 grid with a spacing of 175 μm and 500 representative points. The surfaces were nominally identical, one being obtained from the other by a known rigid transformation. Under comparable conditions, our shape-based method achieved 0.013 μm. This difference perhaps best illustrates the shortcomings of applying 'off-the-shelf' solutions intended for general purpose use or for other specific application areas.

The registration method used in the University of Munich system [30] bears much resemblance to ours, having evidently been developed following a similar line of reasoning. An initial approximation is obtained by identifying three pairs of corresponding points, stable regions are defined by multiple polygons and the disparity function is defined as the sum of squares of point-to-surface distances. Minimisation is by gradient descent, conjugate gradient descent and the Levenberg-Marquardt method [83]. The RMS/point on registered occlusal surfaces was 10.1 μm, mainly due to measurment errors, whereas the intrinsic registration error is described as 'considerably less than 1 μm'.

Least squares minimisation of point-to-surface distances has also been applied to tooth surfaces by Mitchell and Chadwick [31]. Although the system is described as experimental, the reported particulars of its development are especially welcome since they show that the key issues identified by the authors as relevant to the accurate detection of changes in morphology are included within those that have been addressed in this work.

Clinical Applications

The validity of the practical and theoretical methods described above has been confirmed by their successful application in objective clinical research. This section presents examples of some of the types of our investigations which have been enhanced by co-ordinate data analysis.

Wear of Restorations

Quantification of the wear of restored occlusal anterior tooth surfaces has been a dominant area in the study of dental morphology by analysis of co-ordinate data using both CMMs and other measurement systems. Wear over long periods can be readily detectable and since this area has been extensively researched, it did not figure prominently in our investigations. It was of interest, due to the timescales involved, to determine if useful data could be obtained from 'historical' replicas taken for purposes unrelated to co-ordinate acquisition. Figure 25 shows a plane cross-section through a sequence of three replicas of a molar tooth followed longitudinally over a 10-year period taken at 5-year intervals. The restoration covered an area of 80% or more of the occlusal surface of the tooth and extended to one of the approximal surfaces and onto more than half the buccal surface. In the top image, the wear can particularly be seen adjacent to the cavo-surface margin of the restoration, which was more steeply inclined near the area where the restoration meets the tooth surface. The middle image shows the good superposition of the surfaces buccally and lingually, where relatively little wear had occurred, whilst the cusp tips, being related to occlusal contact areas, had worn relatively more. The centre half of the cross-sections shows the greater relative wear of the composite resin restorative material (P-10, 3M Dental Products, St. Paul, Minn., USA). In the lower image the wear at one point on the composite resin material has been quantified and shown to be 345 μm.

Plaque

Plaque is frequently present in sufficient quantity to enable its visual detection from the rendered images (fig. 26). Its distribution can be viewed either on individual cross-sections (fig. 27) or over the entire surface with colour-coded 'subtraction maps' (fig. 28) of the type commonly used in imaging applications [27, 100]. The distribution of plaque is frequently very irregular and therefore measurements of its thickness at individual locations are susceptible to considerable variations. For this reason, plaque thickness is evaluated by permitting the operator of the software to define a rectangular region of interest (usually 1 mm^2) over which the thickness is automatically evaluated at several thousand locations and averaged.

The presence of a stable region required for superposing is ensured by removing the plaque (with gauze) from a region located around the mid-line on the upper coronal half of the tooth prior to replication. Assessment of the methodology is reported by Yeganeh et al. [101, 102]. The method has been applied to compare the plaque removal ability of two toothpastes [103] and proved capable of revealing a statistically significant difference in plaque depth change between the two products (mean = 19 μm, SE = 6.53, $p < 0.01$).

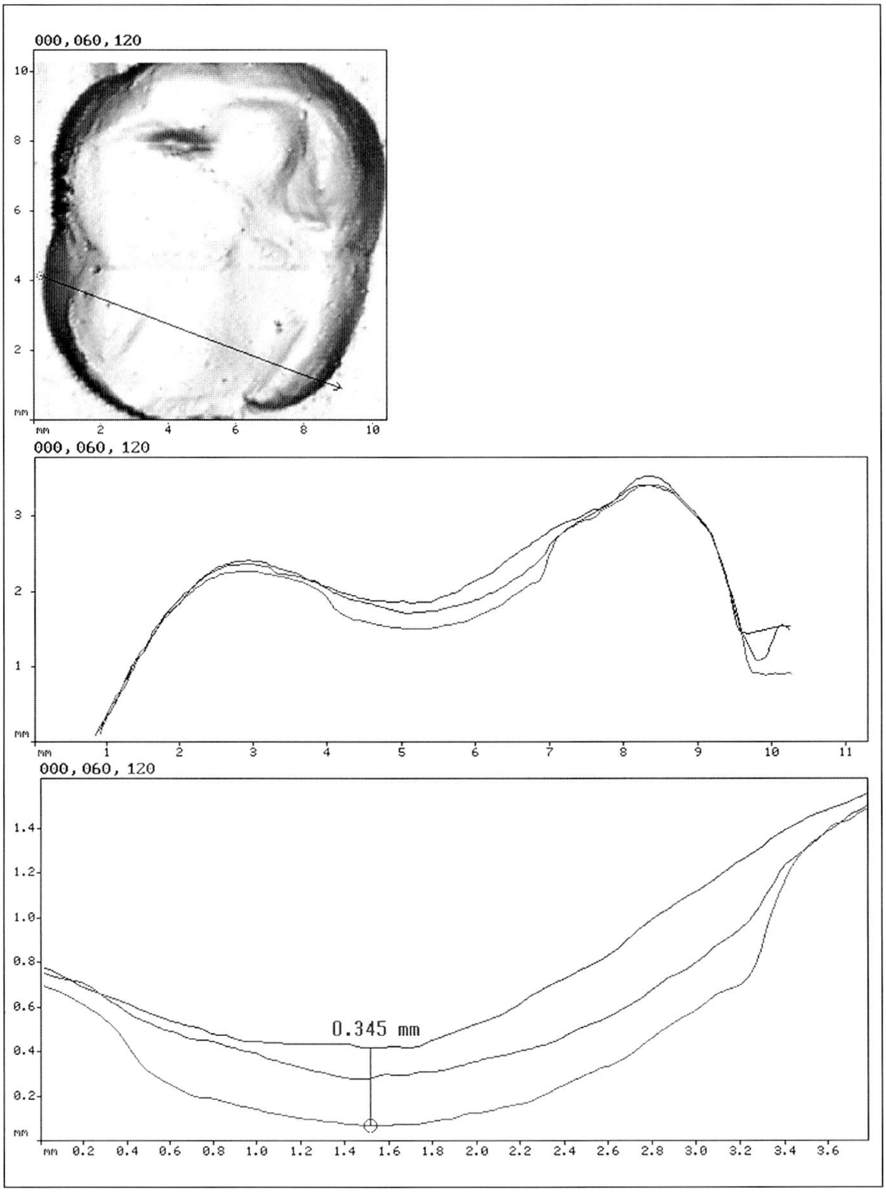

Fig. 25. Wear of a restoration at 5 and 10 years.

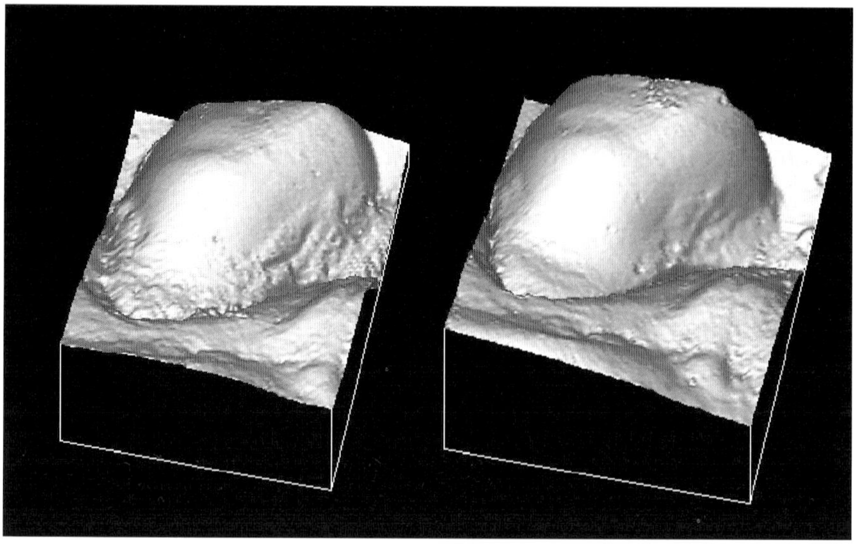

Fig. 26. Plaque before and after cleaning.

Gingivitis

Co-ordinate metrology is particularly well suited to the study of changes in gingival contour, since these are large in relation to the method accuracy and the entire tooth surface can be used as the stable region for superposing. Applications to date include a study of experimentally induced gingivitis over a period of 21 days [104] and canine gingivitis [105].

Effects of Two Toothbrushes on Hard Tissue

The system proved capable of discriminating between the effects of different toothbrushes on hard tissue loss during a 3-month study period, while clinical assessment during the same period did not produce statistically significant observations [106].

Three-Month Assessment of an Antimicrobial Root Sealant

Co-ordinate metrology has previously been used to assess the volume and area of sealant applied to occlusal surfaces [100, 107]. Our system was applied in an investigation of the thickness and wear of a protective root sealant on exposed root surfaces [108]. Impressions were taken before and after the placement of the sealant to assess its thickness (fig. 29) and also after 3 months to assess wear and failure (fig. 30).

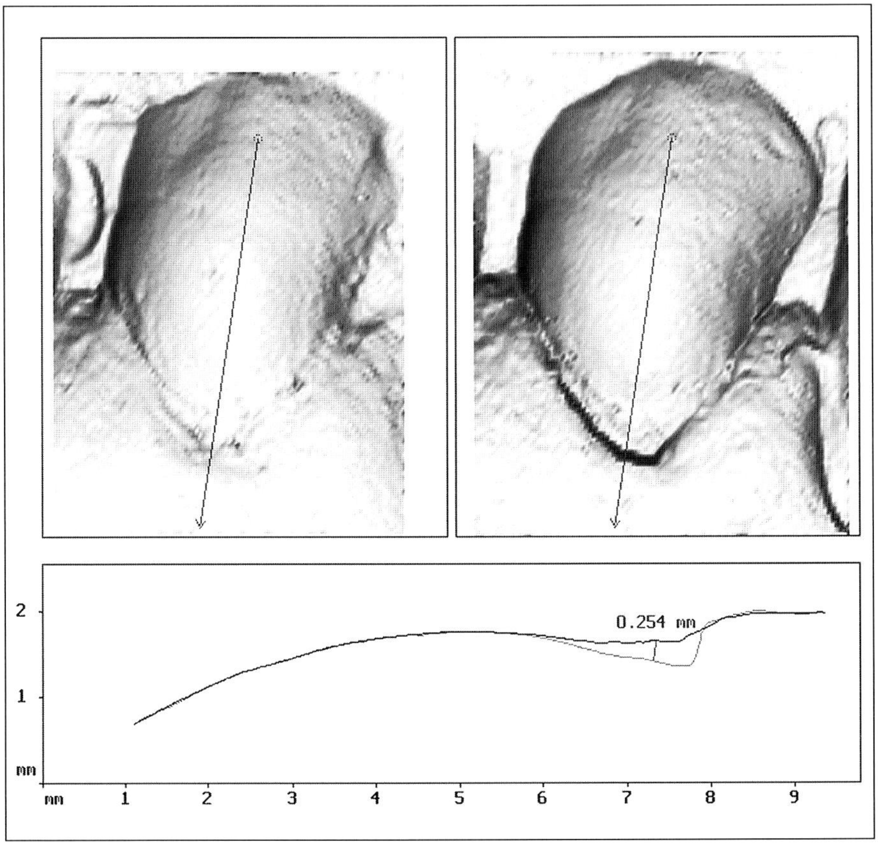

Fig. 27. Plaque cross-section.

Geometry of Crowns and Crown Preparations

The variations in geometry of labial shoulder preparations from a variety of operators and the effects that these variations have on the emergence profile of metal ceramic crowns have been assessed and reported by Seymour et al. [109, 110]. An example is shown in figure 31.

Other Application Areas – Treatment of Inflamed Joints

Replicas of a single inflamed proximal interphalangeal joint injected with a steroid to reduce swelling were made at baseline prior to injection and 2 and 7 days after the steroid injection. The scanning pitch was 300 μm (fig. 32). The RMS/point of stable regions was between 90 and 130 μm – remarkably accurate considering that any bending of the joint would alter the shape

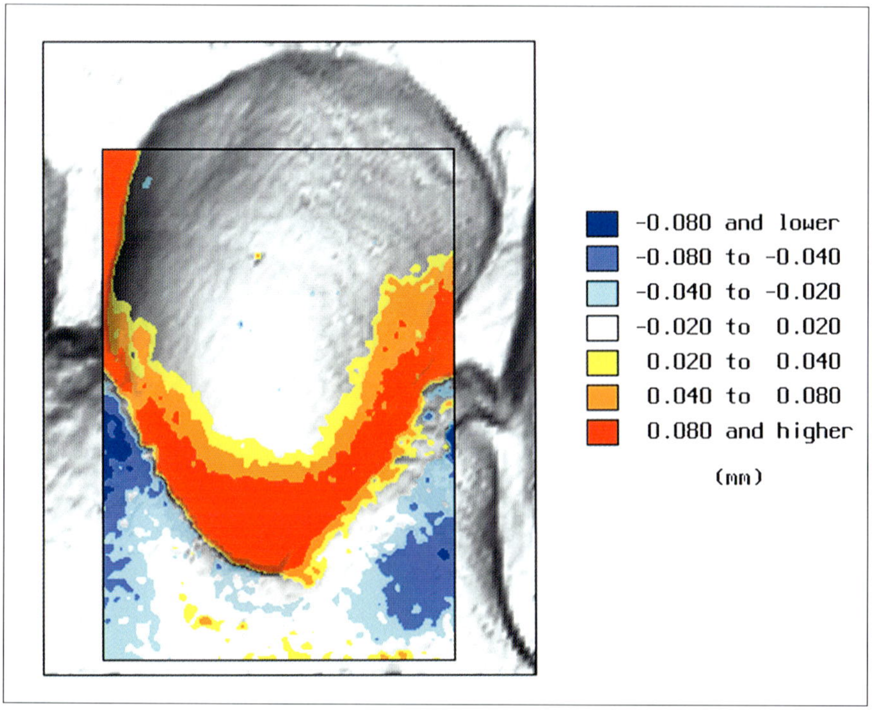

Fig. 28. Plaque-subtraction map.

considerably. The measured improvement (fig. 33) was not detected through clinical observation by the rheumatologist, nor by the patient.

Conclusions

Computer-based methods have in the past been described as 'extremely expensive, subject to superpositioning errors and impractical for evaluating casts in large clinical studies' [22]. With this new system, patient and clinician time consumption is minimal and involves the use of familiar techniques. Since replicas can be obtained easily, speedily and economically, and forwarded to a central laboratory for digitising, the cost implications, even when large clinical studies are involved, are not of the significance that has previously been the case. The replication method is highly repeatable for hard tissue and plaque, less so for soft tisue, but sufficient to permit the reliable detection of changes.

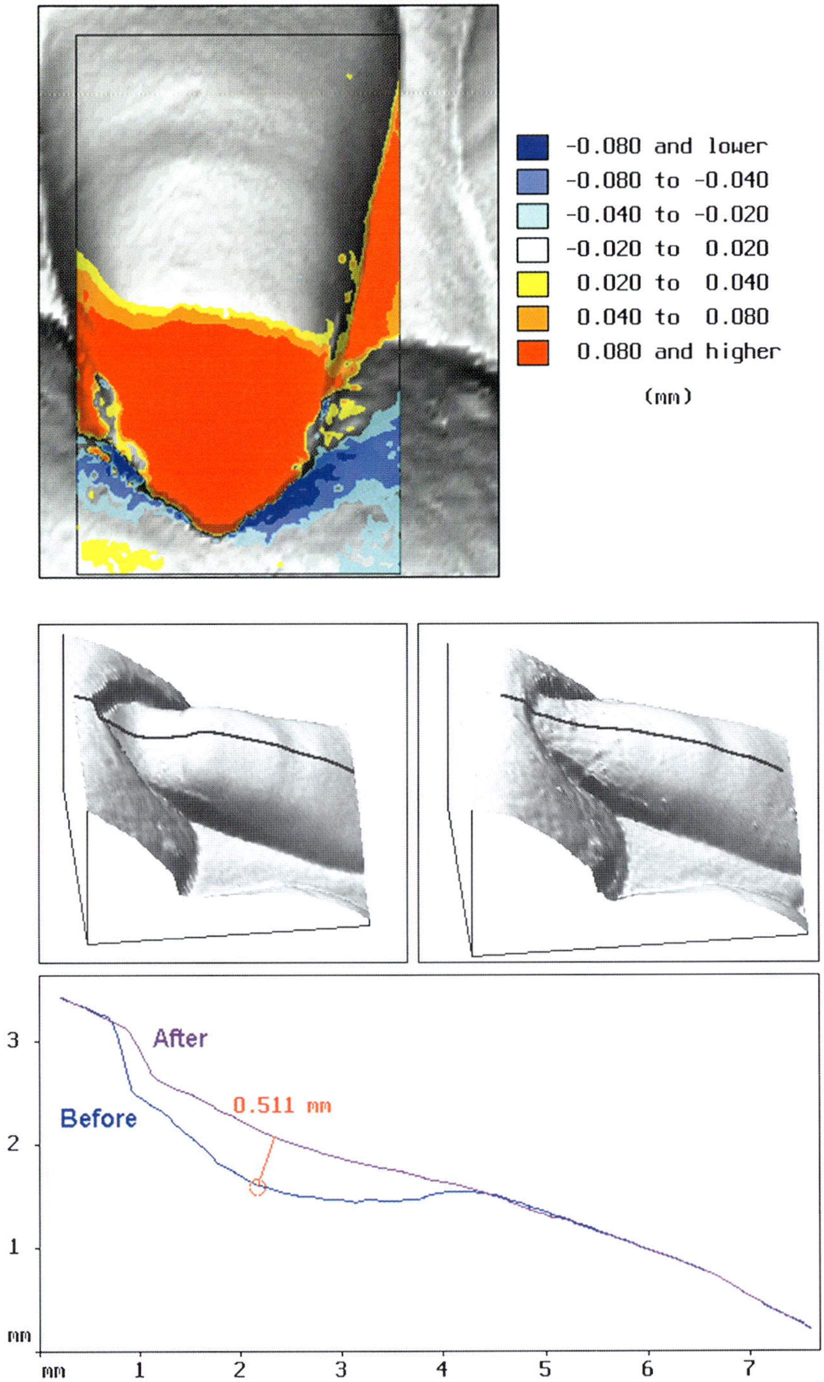

Fig. 29. Extent and depth of applied sealant.

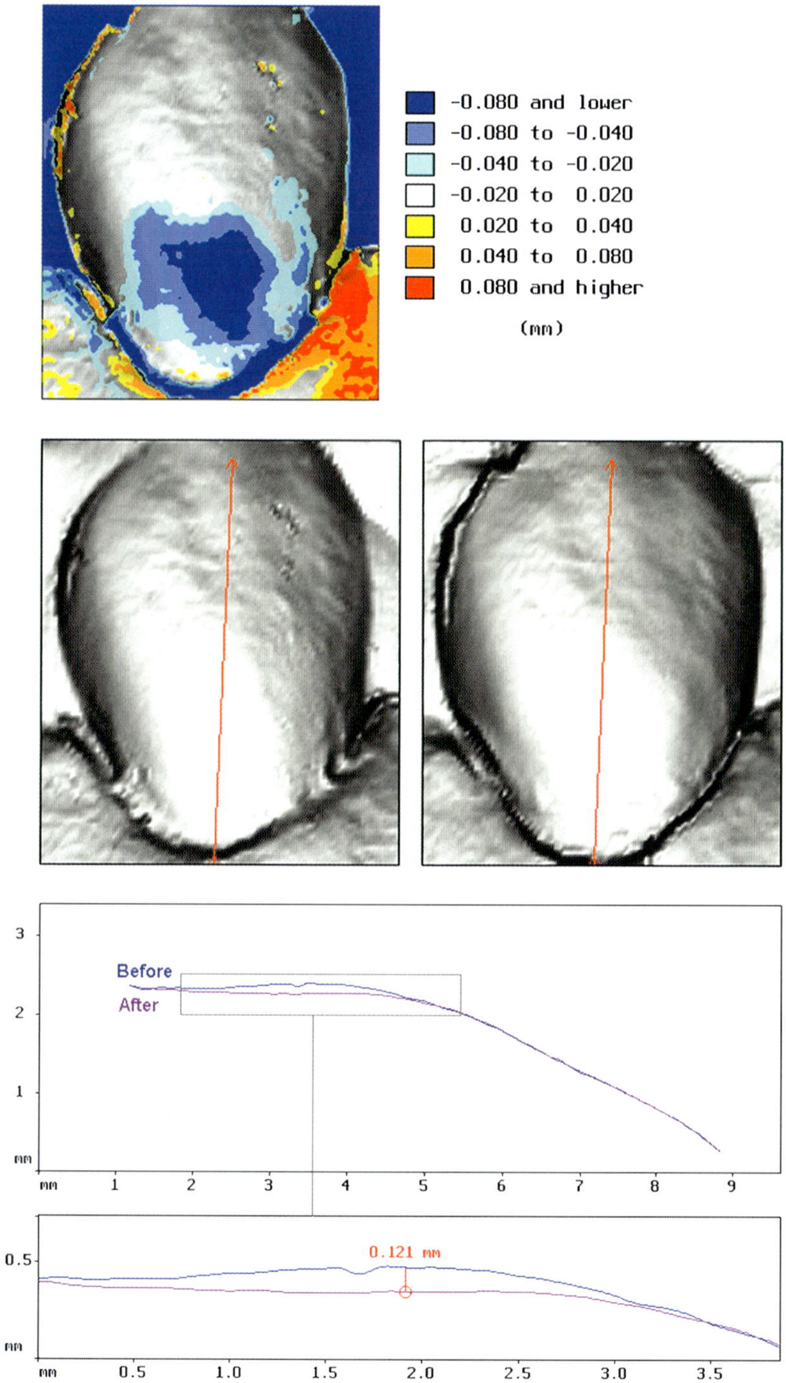

Fig. 30. Sealant wear after 3 months.

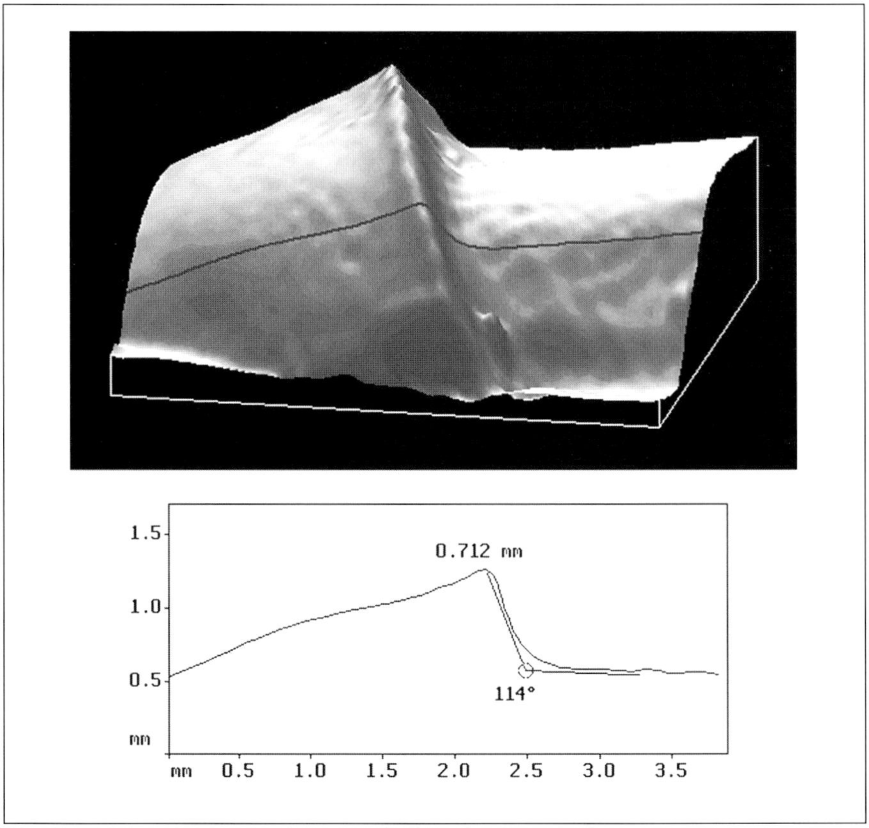

Fig. 31. Geometry of crown preparations.

The majority of co-ordinate data acquisition systems applied in dental research have employed probes which make physical contact with the surface of the specimen. Such probes are not ideal for measuring silicone impressions because they exert pressure which may cause deformation of the elastic impression material and therefore require rigid models to be produced. Additionally, post-processing of the data is necessary to compensate for the shape of the stylus, since the exact point with which it contacts the surface is gradient-dependent [111]. The ability to acquire co-ordinate data directly from standard silicone impressions eliminates the time, effort and potential for additional errors associated with the production of rigid models. The system has been applied over a sufficiently lengthy period to permit a more detailed assessment of its characteristics than has been the case with many other acquisition systems, thus enabling its optimal exploitation.

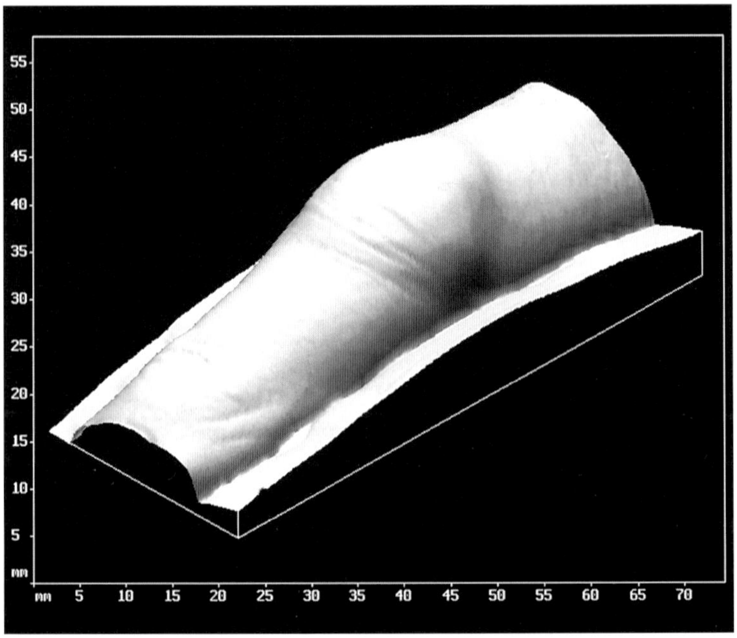

Fig. 32. The surface obtained from a replica of an inflamed joint.

The reference-free superposition of data sets obtained from sequential replicas permits investigations of changes in morphology to be performed which would otherwise be impractical if external markers were required. It can also be applied to replicas and models produced earlier, in studies which have not anticipated the use of co-ordinate metrology.

The registration method itself is based on the well-known principle of least squares optimisation. The convergence has been augmented by Aitken acceleration.

Extensive assessment of the method's accuracy and repeatability on synthetically constructed surfaces and on clinically acquired data has been performed. The registration accuracy of clinically acquired data was found to be 6–9 μm in terms of RMS/point. Operation of the supporting software is straightforward and efficient, requiring little operator training. Its visualisation capabilities permit the creation of images which can be easily perceived and understood by clinicians.

The study and application of co-ordinate data analysis over an extended period has enabled detailed, quantifiable 3-D measurements to be recorded in longitudinal studies on gingivae, plaque and root surfaces of teeth, which

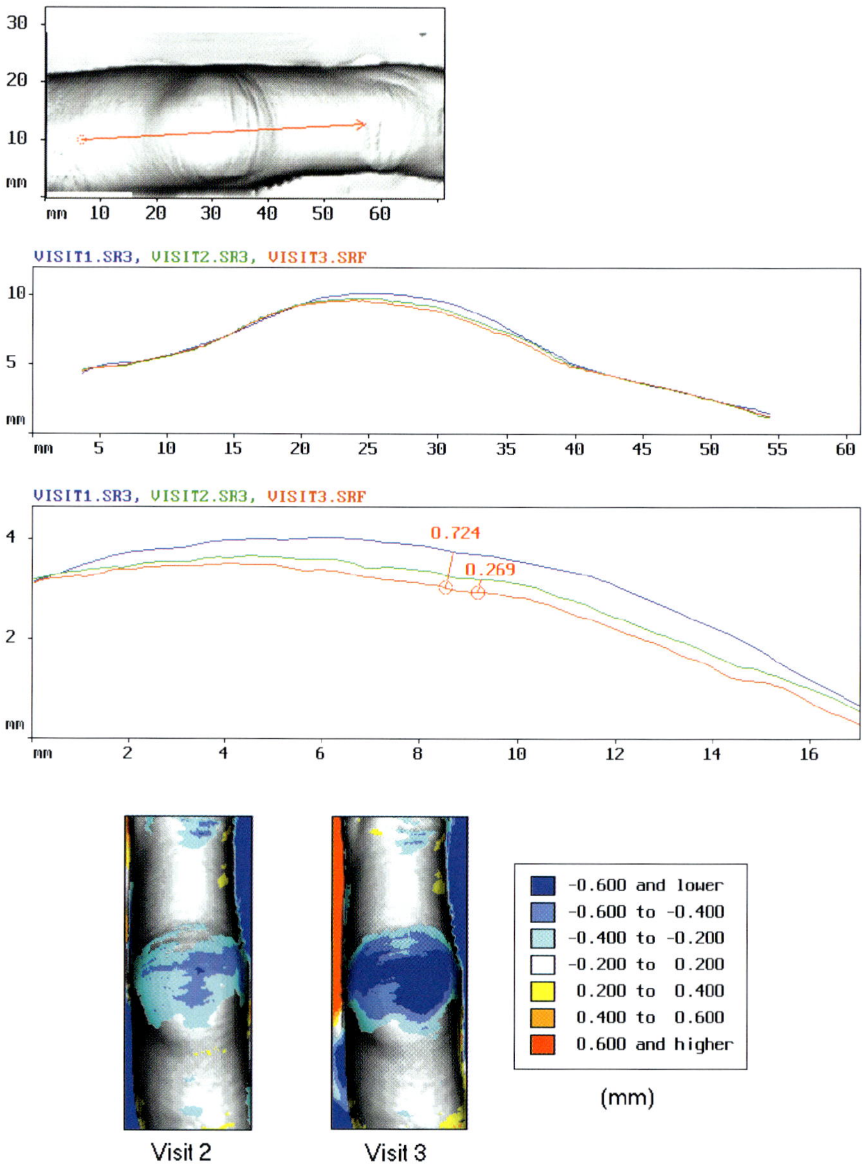

Fig. 33. Progressive improvement relative to baseline.

have been rarely investigated in the past. There is good correlation between the results obtained using the methods described and those determined by clinical examination alone, e.g. plaque indices vs. the measured plaque or changes in gingival contour, though the discriminating power of co-ordinate data analysis is far better. Areas of further clinical research in which the system might be applied are not limited to dentistry, but include a wide category of medical and other investigations of changes in shape.

Acknowledgements

We are grateful to: Prof. Harry Allred, founder of the Dental Metrology Unit; Prof. Maurice Cox of the National Physical Laboratory, for providing mathematical expertise; Mrs Lifong Zou, for digitising all replicas used in these studies; Ms Sharzad Yeganeh, Ms Aylin Baysan, Dr Kevin Seymour and Dr Carolyn Morris-Clapp, clinical investigators, and Prof. David Blake of the University of Bath for collaboration on the study of inflamed joints.

The authors would like to acknowledge the support of clinical studies by: Optiva Corporation, USA; The Scientific Foundation for Dental Diagnosis, Netherlands; Unilever Research, UK; Procter and Gamble, USA; Synthélabo, France and Dentsply, Germany.

References

1 Cvar JF, Ryge G: Criteria for the clinical evaluation of dental restorative materials. USPHS Publication No 790-244. San Francisco, US Government Printing Office, 1971.
2 Leinfelder KF, Taylor DF, Barkmeier WW, Goldberg AJ: Quantitative wear measurement of posterior composite resins. Dent Mater 1986;2:198–201.
3 Elderton RJ: An objective method for measuring the surface morphology of cavities and restorations in vivo. J Oral Rehabil 1977;4:323–334.
4 Chadwick RG, McCabe JF, Walls AW, Mitchell HL, Storer R: Comparison of a novel photogrammetric technique and modified USPHS criteria to monitor the wear of restorations. J Dent 1991;19:39–45.
5 Chadwick RG: Close range photogrammetry – A clinical dental research tool. J Dent 1992;20:235–239.
6 Scott PJ: Pepper's ghost observed in Cape Town. S Afr J Photogram Remote Sensing Cartog 1984;14:89–95.
7 Adams LP, Wilding RJC: Tooth wear measurements using a reflex microscope. J Oral Rehabil 1988;15:605–613.
8 Adams LP, Jooste CH, Thomas CJ: An indirect in vivo method for quantification of wear in denture teeth. Dent Mater 1989;5:31–34.
9 Atkinson JT, Groves D, Lalor MJ, Cunningham J, Williams DF: The measurement of wear in dental restorations using laser dual-source contouring. Wear 1982;76:91–104.
10 Williams DF, Cunningham J, Lalor MJ, Groves D, Atkinson JT: Laser techniques for the evaluation of wear in class II restorations. J Oral Rehabil 1983;10:407–414.
11 Farely DW, Shin D, Jones R, Agrawal CM: The wear of human enamel opposing dental porcelain (abstract). J Dent Res 1999;78:112.
12 Boyde A, Howell PGT, Franc F: Simple SEM stereophotogrammetric method for three-dimensional evaluation of features on flat substrates. J Microsc 1986;143:257–264.

13 Howell PGT, Reid SA: A microcomputer-based system for rapid on-line stereological analysis in the SEM. Scanning 1986;8:139–144.
14 Howell PGT, Boyde A, Ross HF: A three axis stereocomparator for scanning electron microscopic photogrammetry – RS3. Scanning 1986;8:182–186.
15 Anderson P, Davis GR, Elliott JC: Microtomography. Microsc Anal 1994;15:31–33.
16 Nielsen RB, Alyassin AM, Peters DD, Carnes DL, Lancaster J: Microcomputed tomography: An advanced system for detailed endodontic research. J Endod 1995;21:561–568.
17 Balto K, Müller R, Carrington DC, Stashenko P: Quantitation of periapical bone destruction in mice by micro-computed tomography (abstract). J Dent Res 1999;78:122.
18 Watson TF, Boyde A: Confocal light microscopic techniques for examining dental operative procedures and dental materials. Am J Dent 1991;4:193–200.
19 Mörmann WH, Bindl A: The new creativity in ceramic restorations: Dental CAD-CIM. Quintessence Int 1996;27:821–828.
20 Alcañiz M, Chinesta F, Monserrat C, Grau V, Ramón A: An advanced system for the simulation and planning of orthodontic treatments; in Höhne KH, Kikinis R (eds): Visualization in Biomedical Computing. 4th Int Conf. Berlin, Springer, 1996, pp 511–520.
21 Chadwick RG: A review: The assessment of the durability of composite resin restorative materials in vivo. Clin Mater 1989;4:241–253.
22 Bayne SC, Taylor DF, Rekow ED, Wilder AD, Heymann HO: Confirmation of Leinfelder clinical wear standards. Dent Mater 1994;10:11–18.
23 Roulet JF, Reich T, Lutz F: High precision occlusal mapping – A new method for measuring wear of posterior composite resins (abstract). J Dent Res 1983;62:220.
24 Roulet JF: Development of appropriate measuring devices; in Roulet J-F (ed): Degradation of Dental Polymers. Basel, Karger, 1987, pp 101–108.
25 Lambrechts P, Vanherle G, Vuylsteke M, Davidson CL: Quantitative evaluation of the wear resistance of posterior dental restorations. J Dent 1984;12:252–267.
26 DeLong R, Pintado MR, Douglas WH: Measurement of change in surface contour by computer graphics. Dent Mater 1985;1:27–30.
27 Bangerter V, Christensen R, Christensen G: Method for determination of in vivo wear (abstract). J Dent Res 1987;66:126.
28 McDowell GC, Bloem TJ, Lang BR, Asgar K: In vivo wear. Part I: The Michigan computer-graphic measuring system. J Prosthet Dent 1988;60:112–120.
29 Chadwick RG, Mitchell HL, Cameron I, Hunter B, Tulley M: Development of a novel system for assessing tooth and restoration wear. J Dent 1997;25:41–47.
30 Mehl A, Gloger W, Kunzelmann KH, Hickel R: A new optical 3-D device for the detection of wear. J Dent Res 1997;76:1799–1807.
31 Mitchell HL, Chadwick RG: Mathematical shape matching as a tool in tooth wear assessment – Development and conduct. J Oral Rehabil 1998;15:921–928.
32 Jovanovski V, Tay WM, Zou L, Anderson IJ, Cox MG, Forbes AB, Allred H, Morganstein SI, Lynch E: Objective assessment of three-dimensional structures in clinical dentistry using methods of co-ordinate metrology. Nanobiology 1996;4:55–61.
33 Starcke EN Jr: A historical review of complete denture impression materials. J Am Dent Assoc 1975;91:1037–1041.
34 Doubleday B: Impression materials. Br J Orthod 1998;25:133–140.
35 Chee WW, Donovan TE: Polyvinyl siloxane impression materials: A review of properties and techniques. J Prosthet Dent 1992;68:728–732.
36 Fano V, Gennari PU, Ortalli I: Dimensional stability of silicone-based impression materials. Dent Mater 1992;8:105–109.
37 Clancy JM, Scandrett FR, Ettinger RL: Long-term dimensional stability of three current elastomers. J Oral Rehabil 1983;10:325–333.
38 Williams PT, Jackson DG, Bergman W: An evaluation of the time-dependent dimensional stability of eleven elastomeric impression materials. J Prosthet Dent 1984;52:120–125.
39 Tjan AH, Whang SB, Tjan AH, Sarkissian R: Clinically oriented evaluation of the accuracy of commonly used impression materials. J Prosthet Dent 1986;56:4–8.

40 Corso M, Abanomy A, Di Canzio J, Zurakowski D, Morgano SM: The effect of temperature changes on the dimensional stability of polyvinyl siloxane and polyether impression materials. J Prosthet Dent 1998;79:626–631.
41 Dastane A, Vaidyanthan TK, Vaidyanthan J, Mehra R, Hesby R: Development and evaluation of a new 3-D digitization and computer graphic system to study the anatomic tissue and restoration surfaces. J Oral Rehabil 1996;23:25–34.
42 Zou L, Yang QP, Jovanovski V, Tay WM, Lynch E: Measurement of tooth morphology using a laser probe fitted on a co-ordinate measuring machine; in De Chiffre L (ed): Proc 4th Int IMEKO Symp on Laser Metrology for Precision Measurement and Inspection in Industry. Lyngby, Center for Geometrical Metrology, Institute of Manufacturing Engineering, Technical University of Denmark, 1996, pp 11–20.
43 Zou L, Jovanovski V, Tay WM, Lynch E: Error distribution on a digitised datum sphere (abstract). J Dent Res 1996;75:1165.
44 Zou L, Jovanovski V, Tay WM, Lynch E: The influence of three parameters on laser probe scanning of irregular surfaces (abstract). J Dent Res 1995;74:895.
45 Faux ID, Pratt MJ: Computational Geometry for Design and Manufacture. Chichester, Ellis Horwood, 1979.
46 Catley D, Whittle C, Thornton P: Applications of the general surface definition and manipulation system GENSURF; in Martin RR (ed): The Mathematics of Surfaces II. Oxford, Clarendon Press, 1987, pp 171–202.
47 Sarkar B, Menq C-H: Smooth-surface approximation and reverse engineering. Computer Aided Design 1991;23:623–628.
48 Weir DJ, Milroy MJ, Bradley C, Vickers GW: Reverse engineering physical models employing wrap-around B-spline surfaces and quadrics. Proc Inst Mech Eng [B] 1996;210:147–157.
49 McLain DH: Drawing contours from arbitrary data points. Computer J 1976;17:318–324.
50 MacCarthy BL, Handscomb DC: The approximation of hydrographic survey data using tensor-product B-spline surfaces; in Handscomb DC (ed): The Mathematics of Surfaces III. Oxford, Clarendon Press, 1989, pp 373–389.
51 Ateshian GA: A B-spline least-squares surface-fitting method for articular surfaces or diarthroidal joints. J Biomech Eng 1993;115:366–373.
52 Cox MG: Practical spline approximation; in Turner PR (ed): Lecture Notes in Mathematics 965: Topics in Numerical Analysis. Berlin, Springer, 1982, pp 79–112.
53 Cox MG: Algorithms for Spline Curves and Surfaces. NPL Report DITC 166/90. Teddington, National Physical Laboratory, 1990.
54 de Boor C: A Practical Guide to Splines. New York, Springer, 1978.
55 Cox MG: The numerical evaluation of B-splines. J Inst Math Appl 1972;10:134–149.
56 de Boor C: On calculating with B-splines. J Approx Theory 1972;6:50–62.
57 Sabin MA: Contouring – The state of the art; in Earnshaw RA (ed): Fundamental Algorithms for Computer Graphics. NATO ASI Series, vol F17. Berlin, Springer, 1985, pp 411–482.
58 Anderson IJ, Cox MG, Mason JC: Tensor-product spline interpolation to data on or near a family of lines. Numer Alg 1993;5:193–204.
59 Anderson IJ, Mason JC: Surface fitting by exploiting data distribution; in Mullineux G (ed): Mathematics of Surfaces VI. Oxford, Clarendon Press, 1996, pp 137–152.
60 Anderson IJ: A piecewise approach to piecewise approximation. Numer Alg 1997;15:132–152.
61 Anderson IJ, Pink CK: Spline surface fitting of rank deficient problems: A natural solution; in Goodman T, Martin R (eds): The Mathematics of Surfaces VII. Winchester, Information Geometers, 1997, pp 439–461.
62 Gouraud H: Continuous shading of curved surfaces. IEEE Trans Comp [C] 1971;20:623–628.
63 Heap BR, Pink MG: Three contouring algorithms. NPL Mathematical Report 81. Teddington, National Physical Laboratory, 1969.
64 Schumaker LL: Fitting surfaces to scattered data; in Lorentz GG, Chui CK, Schumaker LL (eds): Approximation Theory II. New York, Academic Press, 1976, pp 203–268.
65 DeLong R, Bramwell MC: Matching an initial surface to a worn surface subject to rotation and translation; in Martin RR (ed): The Mathematics of Surfaces II. Oxford, Clarendon Press, 1987, pp 137–149.

66 Mirsky L: An Introduction to Linear Algebra. Oxford, Clarendon Press, 1995.
67 Schreier O, Sperner E: Modern Algebra and Matrix Theory. New York, Chelsea Press, 1951.
68 Schwerdtfeger H: Introduction to Linear Algebra and the Theory of Matrices. Groningen, Noordhoff, 1950.
69 Hanson RJ, Norris MJ: Analysis of measurements based on the singular value decomposition. SIAM J Sci Stat Comp 1981;2:363–373.
70 Arun KS, Huang TS, Blostein SD: Least-squares fitting of two 3-D point sets. IEEE Trans Pattern Anal Machine Intell 1987;9:698–700.
71 Kanatani K: Analysis of 3-D rotation fitting. IEEE Trans Pattern Anal Machine Intell 1994;16: 543–549.
72 Horn BKP: Closed-form solution of absolute orientation using unit quaternions. J Opt Soc Am 1987;4:629–642.
73 Benjemaa R, Schmitt F: A solution for the registration of multiple 3D point sets using unit quaternions; in Burkhardt H, Neumann B (eds): Computer Vision – ECCV '98. Berlin, Springer, 1998, vol 2, pp 241–254.
74 Golub GH, Van Loan CF: Matrix Computations, ed 2. London, Johns Hopkins University Press, 1989.
75 Press WH, Teukolsky SA, Vetterling WT, Flannery BP: Numerical Recipes in C, ed 2. Cambridge, Cambridge University Press, 1992.
76 Bartlett DW, Smith BGN: Measurment of tooth wear in patients with palatal erosion. Br Dent J 1997;182:179–184.
77 Arai K, Fujita M, Ishikawa H: Recording of casts in ICP with an optical 3D measuring system (abstract). J Dent Res 1999;78:162.
78 Bloem TJ, McDowell GC, Lang BR, Powers JM: In vivo wear. Part II: Wear and abrasion of composite restorative materials. J Prosthet Dent 1988;60:242-249.
79 Toennies KD, Udupa JK, Herman GT, Wornom IL, Buchman SR: Registration of 3D objects and surfaces. IEEE Comput Graphics Appl 1990;10:52–62.
80 Bedford J, Zou L, Jovanovski V, Lynch E: Reproducibility of data collected by a co-ordinate measuring machine (abstract). J Dent Res 1993;72:742.
81 Jovanovski V, Zou L, Tay WM, Lynch E, Cox MG: Superposition of co-ordinate data obtained from a sequence of replicas (abstract). J Dent Res 1995;74:895.
82 Jovanovski V, Zou L, Tay WM, Lynch E, Cox MG: Assessment of three-dimensional structures in clinical dentistry; in Ciarlini P, Cox MG, Pavese F, Richter D (eds): Advanced Mathematical Tools in Metrology III. Singapore, World Scientific, 1997, pp 263–265.
83 Gill PE, Murray W, Wright MH: Practical Optimization. London, Academic Press, 1981.
84 Anderson IJ, Turner DA, Mason JC: An efficient algorithm for solving the surface foot point problem; in Cripps R (ed): The Mathematics of Surfaces VIII. Winchester, Information Geometers, 1998, pp 89–103.
85 Grimson WEL, Ettinger GJ, White SJ, Lozano-Pérez T, Wells WM, Kikinis R: An automatic registration method for frameless stereotaxy, image guided surgery and enhanced reality visualization. IEEE Trans Med Imaging 1996;15:129–140.
86 Ellis RE, Fleet DJ, Bryant JT, Rudan J, Fenton P: A method for evaluating CT-based surgical registration; in Troccaz J, Grimson E, Mösges R (eds): Proc CVRMED-MRCAS '97. Berlin, Springer, 1997, pp 141–150.
87 Pennec X, Thirion J-P: Validation of 3-D Registration Methods based on Points and Frames. INRIA Report 2470. Sophia-Antipolis, INRIA, 1995.
88 Simon DA, Kanade T: Geometric constraint analysis and synthesis: Methods for improving shape-based registration accuracy; in Troccaz J, Grimson E, Mösges R (eds): Proc CVRMED-MRCAS '97. Berlin, Springer, 1997,pp 181–190.
89 Stoddart AJ, Lemke S, Hilton A, Renn T: Estimating pose uncertainty for surface registration. Image Vision Comput 1998;16:111–120.
90 van den Elsen P, Pol E-JD, Viergever MA: Medical image matching – A review with classification. IEEE Engineering Med Biol Mag 1993;12:26–39.
91 Lavalée S: Registration for computer-integrated surgery: Methodology, state of the art; in Taylor RH (ed): Computer-Integrated Surgery. Cambridge, MIT Press, 1995, pp 77–97.

92 Besl PJ, McKay ND: A method for registration of 3-D shapes. IEEE Trans Pattern Anal Machine Intell 1992;14:239–256.
93 Chen Y, Medioni G: Object modeling by registration of multiple range images. Image Vision Computing 1992;10:145–155.
94 Pelizzari CA, Chen GTY, Spelbring DR, Weichselbaum RR, Chen C-T: Accurate three-dimensional registration of CT, PET and/or MR images of the brain. J Comput Assist Tomogr 1989;13:20–26.
95 Pelizzari CA, Tan KK, Levin DN, Chen GTY, Balter J: Interactive 3D patient-image registration; in Colchester ACF, Hawkes DJ (eds): Information Processing in Medical Imaging, 12th International Conference. Berlin, Springer, 1991, pp 132–141.
96 Walsh GR: Methods of Optimisation. London, Wiley, 1975.
97 DeLong R, Douglas WH: An artificial oral environment for testing dental materials. IEEE Trans Biomed Eng 1991;38:339–345.
98 DeLong R, Pintado MR, Heinzen M, Ko CC, Douglas WH: A comparison of contact and optical methods for measuring abfraction wear (abstract). J Dent Res 1999;78:161.
99 DeLong R, Pintado MR, Douglas WH, Taylor J, Breuer MM: Quantification of clinical changes in the gingival crest height using computer graphics (abstract). J Dent Res 1993;72:330.
100 Pintado MR, Conry JP, Douglas WH: Measurement of sealant volume in vivo using image-processing technology. Quintessence Int 1988;19:613–617.
101 Yeganeh S, Zou L, Jovanovski V, Heath MR, Lynch E: Objective quantification of plaque thickness in vivo (abstract). J Dent Res 1996;75:84.
102 Yeganeh S, Lynch E, Jovanovski V, Zou L: Quantification of root surface plaque using a new 3-D laser scanning method. J Clin Periodontol 1999;26:692–697.
103 Waterfield PC, Shearer B, Lynch E, Jovanovski V, Morris-Clapp C: Metrology: A novel method to measure plaque removal by dentifrices (abstract). J Dent Res 1999;78:498.
104 Yeganeh S, Lynch E, Shearer B, Heath MR, Jovanovski V, Zou L: Clinical and metrology assessment of experimentally induced gingivitis (abstract). J Dent Res 1999;78:351.
105 Snider A, Buchanan W, Yeh C, Donovan Brand R, Mahony L, Jovanovski V, Zou L, Lynch E: Canine gingivitis assessment by computer aided 3 dimensional ccordinate metrology (abstract). J Dent Res 1999;78:351.
106 Savill G, Grigor J, Huntingdon E, Jackson R, Lynch E: Toothbrush design: Adapting for the future. Int Dent J 1998;48:519–525.
107 Conry JP, Pintado MR, Douglas WH: Measurement of fissure sealant surface area by computer. Quintessence Int 1990;21:27–33.
108 Baysan A, Lynch E, Jovanovski V, Brailsford S, Zou L, Beighton D: Three month assessment of an antimicrobial root sealant (abstract). J Dent Res 1999;78:444.
109 Seymour K, Zou L, Samarawickrama DYD, Lynch E: Assessment of shoulder dimensions and angles of porcelain bonded to metal crown preparations. J Prosthet Dent 1996;75:406–411.
110 Seymour KG: Variations in the Labial 'Shoulder' Geometry of Teeth Prepared to Receive Metal Ceramic Crowns; PhD thesis, University of London, 1998.
111 Hewlett ER, Orro ME, Clark GT: Accuracy testing of three-dimensional digitizing systems. Dent Mater 1992;8:49–53.

Dr. Vladimir Jovanovski, Department of Adult Oral Health,
St. Bartholomew's and the Royal London School of Medicine and Dentistry,
Turner Street, London E1 2AD (UK)
Tel. +44 20 7377 7000/ext. 2118, Fax +44 20 7377 7375, E-Mail V.Jovanovski@mds.qmw.ac.uk

Faller RV (ed): Assessment of Oral Health.
Monogr Oral Sci. Basel, Karger, 2000, vol 17, pp 130–143

Objective Quantification of Plaque Using Digital Image Analysis

Paul A. Sagel, Phillipe G. Lapujade, Joseph M. Miller, Richard J. Sunberg

Procter & Gamble Company, Health Care Research Center, Mason, Ohio, USA

Abstract

Dental plaque is the precursor to many oral diseases (e.g. gingivitis, periodontitis, caries) and thus its removal and control are an important aspect of oral hygiene. Many of the oral care products available today remove or inhibit the growth of dental plaque. Historically, the antiplaque efficacy of products was measured in blinded clinical trials where the amount of plaque on teeth is assessed via subjective visual grading with predefined scales such as the Turesky index. The ability of the examiner to consistently apply the index over time and the sensitivity of the scales often leads to large, expensive clinical trials. The present invention is an automatic measurement of plaque coverage on the facial surfaces of teeth using a digital image analysis technique. Dental plaque disclosed with fluorescein is digitally imaged under long-wave ultraviolet light. Ultraviolet illumination of fluorescein-disclosed plaque produces an image where the pixels of the image can be categorically classified based on color into one of five classes: teeth; plaque; gingiva; plaque on gingiva, or lip retractors. The amount of plaque on teeth can be determined by summation of the number of plaque pixels. The percent coverage is calculated from the number of plaque pixels and teeth pixels in the image. The digital image analysis of plaque allows facial plaque levels to be precisely measured (RSD = 3.77%). In application, the digital image analysis of plaque is capable of measuring highly significant plaque growth inhibition of a stannous fluoride dentifrice with as few as 10 subjects in a cross-over design.

Introduction

Dental plaque is the precursor to many oral diseases (e.g. gingivitis, periodontitis, caries) and thus its removal and control are an important aspect of oral hygiene [1]. In the simplest sense, plaque is comprised of bacterial masses on the surface of teeth, usually occurring at the gingival margin and in the interproximal areas. To the eye, plaque appears as a white gelatinous mass which can easily be removed with a toothbrush. Plaque continually left in a particular area may calcify and become tartar which requires dental scaling for removal. One of the purposes of marketed and developmental oral care products, such as toothbrushes, dentifrice and interdental aids, is to provide plaque removal or inhibition of plaque growth. The plaque efficacy of the agents and devices is evaluated using a variety of in vitro, ex vivo and in vivo techniques [2–8]. The majority of the in vivo measurement techniques are based upon a trained expert's subjective assessment of the amount of plaque on teeth. Two common indices used to assess plaque levels are the modified Turesky and Silness-Loe [1, 2].

The modified Turesky index is a 0–5 integer assessment of the plaque on labial, buccal and lingual surfaces of each individual tooth [3]. The plaque is visualized by staining the plaque with a disclosing agent. The most commonly used agent is erythrosin, marketed under the name Red Coat®. This technique is widely used to evaluate the antiplaque efficacy of many toothbrushes, rinses and dentifrices [3].

The Silness-Loe technique [1, 2] is a 0–2 integer scale based on visual and probing assessments of plaque to determine coverage and thickness. Typically, Silness-Loe does not involve the use of plaque-disclosing agents.

The subjective indices are limited for two primary reasons:

(1) Inconsistent application of the index, especially in long clinical trials, often leads to greater variation in the data. To account for the variability, larger numbers of subjects are involved in the studies. The end result is higher cost and more complex clinical studies. Most plaque clinical studies involve at least 20 subjects per treatment group and sometimes exceed 50 depending upon the magnitude of the plaque benefit the agent or device delivers relative to controls.

(2) Sensitivity of the scale often leads to larger studies required to define averages. For example, if a particular tooth area is assessed as a Turesky index of 1 and a tooth brush removes 50% of the plaque at this site, the resultant Turesky index is still 1. In order for the index to be 0, the plaque must be completely removed. The subjective indices attempt to account for this by using a nonlinear scale with plaque coverage [3].

Development of Automated Plaque Area Measurement

An objective measure of plaque coverage on teeth would eliminate several challenges associated with using subjective grading techniques. The main ad-

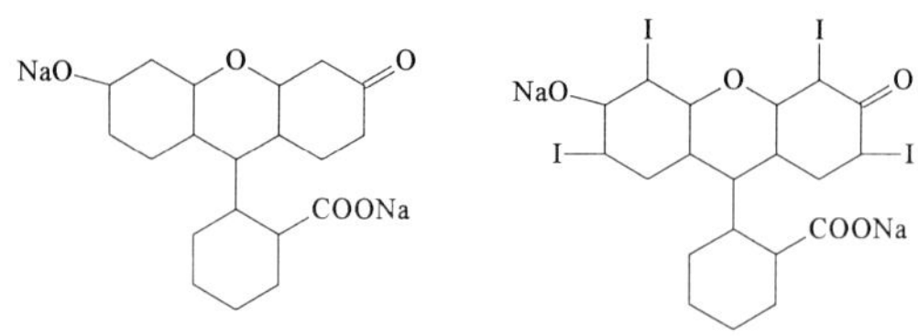

Fig. 1. Chemical structure of Red Coat and fluorescein.

vantages are the consistency of grading throughout trials, smaller clinical trials and no need for a trained expert. Early attempts to develop objective plaque measures included sampling and weighing the plaque mass [4] and photography of disclosed plaque followed by tracing the plaque areas with tracing paper and area calculation of plaque cutouts [5]. Neither technique has proven useful due to the inherent problems associated with sampling all of the plaque and the amount of time associated with tracing and cutting out plaque pictures.

The development of the digital camera coupled with image analysis software yielded the first attempts to develop an imaging system capable of capturing pictures of disclosed plaque and automated measurement of plaque coverage. The first attempts utilized a red coat-disclosing agent and did not enable the analysis software to distinguish between plaque on the teeth, gingival plaque and gingiva due to the close red color of the three entities.

A fluorescein plaque-disclosing agent provides the solution to problems associated with using Red Coat. Fluorescein, FD&C yellow No. 8, is a UV fluorescent dye that absorbs into dental plaque in a fashion very similar to Red Coat. Previous studies have shown that fluorescein and Red Coat disclose plaque in a similar fashion, not surprising considering the chemical structural similarity between Red Coat and fluorescein [9, 10] (fig. 1).

Under long wave UV light, fluorescein produces a disclosed plaque on teeth that is significantly different from the color of gingival tissue and gingival plaque. Plaque on teeth fluoresces yellow, plaque on gingiva fluoresces green, teeth fluoresce blue and gingiva are nearly black. These unique properties of fluorescein make it an excellent candidate for automatic determination of plaque coverage by computer-aided imaging using color as the classifying feature. Figure 2 is an example of fluorescein-disclosed plaque imaged under UV light. Note the color separation between the plaque on the teeth and the plaque on the gingiva.

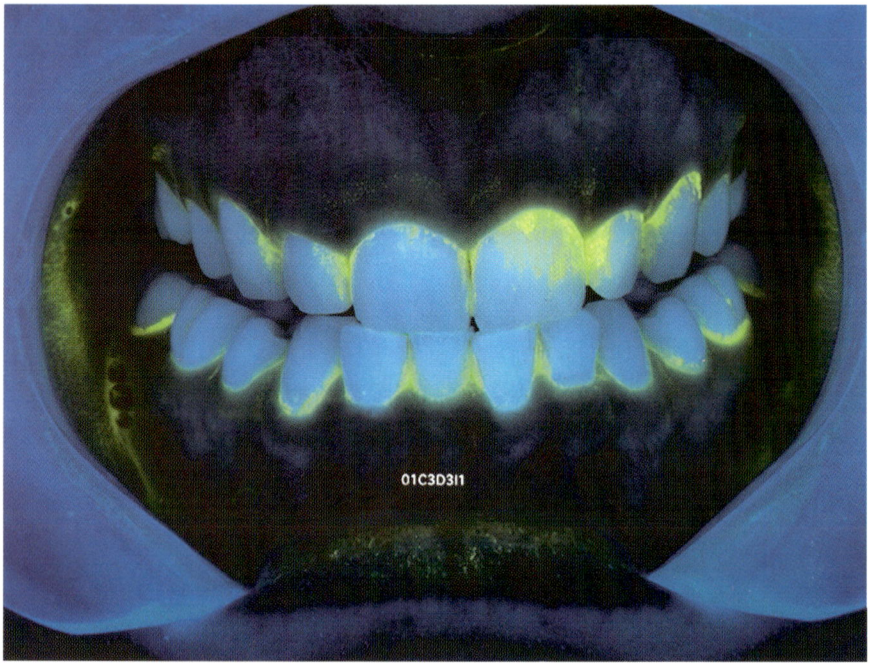

Fig. 2. Fluorescein-disclosed plaque photographed under UV light.

The five distinct classes under UV light, plaque on the teeth, plaque on the gingiva, teeth, gums and lip retractors, are separated by at least 50 color values (255 maximum) in red, green, blue (RGB) color space. The average color values for the classes are shown in table 1.

Generalized Approach to Quantitative Measurement of in vivo Plaque

The wide color separation of fluorescein-disclosed UV images of plaque allows a relatively simple procedure known as the least squared distance discriminant classification to be used to automatically quantify plaque area on teeth. Each pixel (smallest picture element) of an image can be classified as plaque on teeth, plaque on gingiva, teeth, gingiva or lip retractors. After classification and summation of the total number of pixels in each class, the percent plaque coverage can be calculated from the following:

$$(\%\ \text{Plaque on teeth}) = \frac{(\text{number of pixels of plaque on teeth})}{(\text{number of pixels of plaque on teeth}) + (\text{number of pixels of teeth})}.$$

Table 1. Average red, green and blue values for classes

Class	Red	Green	Blue
Plaque on teeth	89.4	208.5	54.8
Plaque on gingiva	52.1	147.6	27.6
Gingiva	13.3	57.9	28.4
Teeth	40.7	137.1	123.2
Lip Retractors	10.7	79.8	135.3

Least Squared Distance Calculations

Pixel classification is accomplished by calculating the scalar distance in RGB color space from the pixel to be classified to the median RGB color of each predefined class. The pixel is classified in the group to which the scalar distance is least. The mathematical procedure is outlined in the Appendix.

Physical System

UV images of disclosed plaque are captured with a Fujix 1000 CCD camera controlled by a high-end PC of 200 MHz or better. Light is supplied by two Balcar long-wave UV flashes, model FX-60, equipped with cutoff filters at 265 nm. The flashes are powered by Balcar 2400 power packs and controlled by the PC as well. To avoid damage to the subject's eyes, UV-filtering glasses are worn. The system is set up with one flash head on each side of the camera at a 45° angle with the subject as shown in figure 3.

The subject's chin is placed in a fixed chin cup mounted 45.5 cm from the camera lens as shown in figure 4. Lip retractors are used to allow uniform lighting of the teeth and obtain unobstructed images. To ensure good subject positioning, a live image is displayed on a positioning monitor. Once a good position is established, a UV image is captured and a reference position image is stored according to subject identification number. At subsequent visits, the stored positioning images are used to realign the subjects to the same position. Repositioning is accomplished by overlaying a live image on top of the stored image. The subject's position is adjusted so that the live image overlays the stored image. This is accomplished with a video-blending system capable of displaying a live image superimposed on a stored image.

System Calibration and Image Color Correction

The imaging system is calibrated using color charts. After warming up the system, an image of a color chart is captured. The color chart contains sixteen 1×1 cm color chips. The color values are extracted from the image

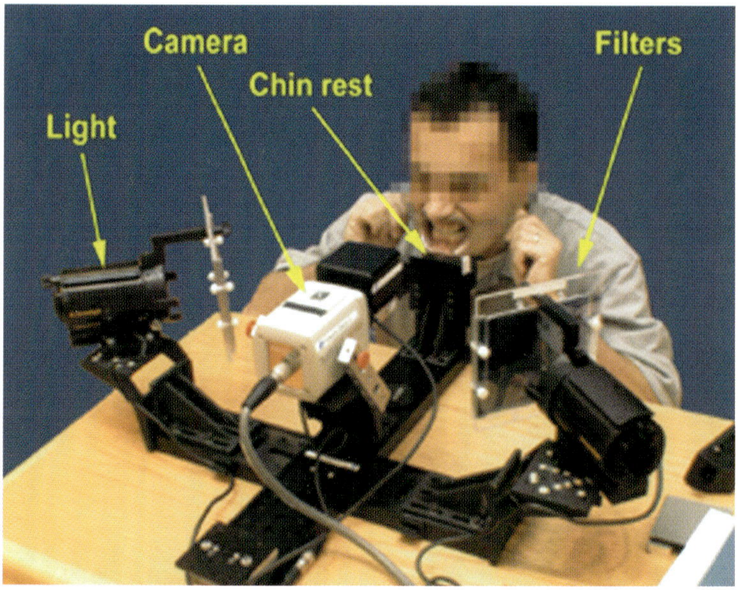

Fig. 3. Physical setup of system for capturing images.

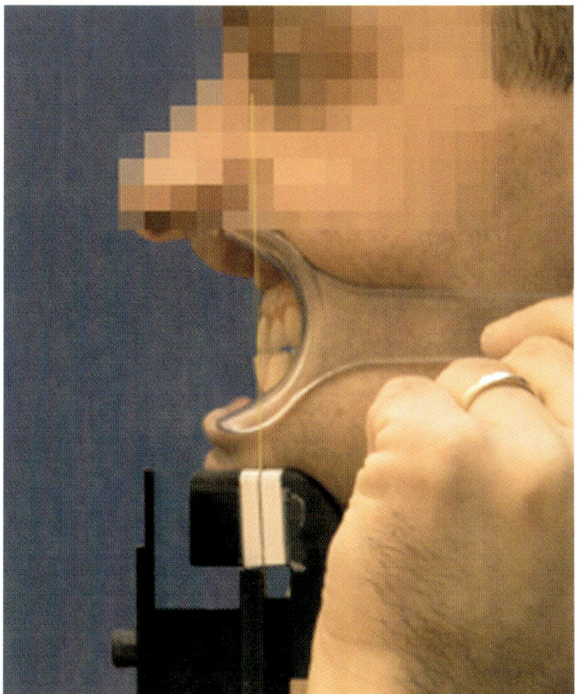

Fig. 4. Chin rest.

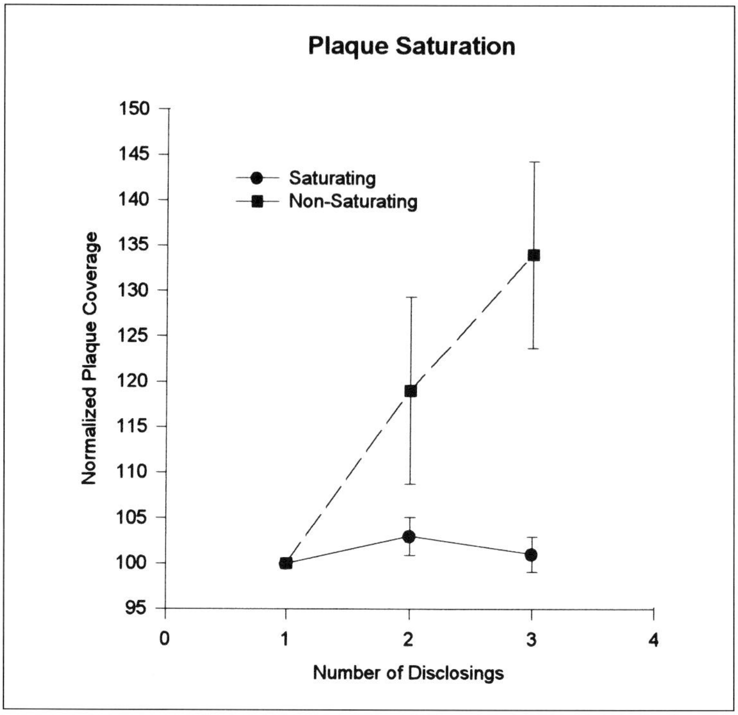

Fig. 5. Plaque saturation with fluorescein.

and compared to a standard image of the color chart. Based on the differences between the captured chart and the standard chart, a color correction is generated to correct images for the small variations of the camera and lighting configuration. The color correction is a polynomial regression between color values in the captured image and the standard color values. Each pixel in the image receives a color correction to its RGB values based on this regression. If large differences exist ($>5\%$ differences), the system setup is adjusted to account for the problem (e.g. increase lighting intensity, adjust camera white balance, etc.).

Disclosing Plaque with Fluorescein

Disclosing plaque is not trivial when using a precise measurement technique such as the digital image analysis. Insufficient disclosing of the plaque results in underestimated plaque levels. A simple technique for determining the adequacy of plaque disclosing is a series of disclosing and measurement to ensure constant plaque levels. Figure 5 summarizes the results of two plaque-

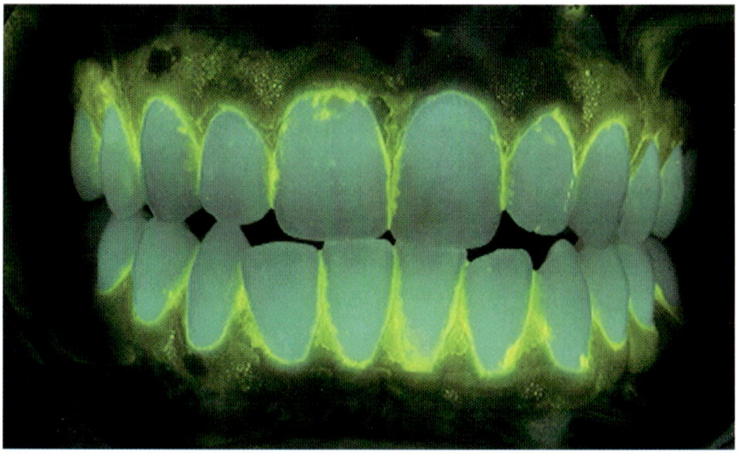

Fig. 6. Actual image.

disclosing techniques in which one disclosing procedure does not fully saturate the plaque and the second procedure fully discloses the plaque. For ease of comparison, the initial plaque levels are normalized to 100%. Subsequent measures are then expressed as percent of initial plaque levels. Thus, a saturating disclosing procedure will maintain 100% of the initial level and unsaturating procedures will show more than 100% after several disclosings. Notice how the plaque area increases with multiple disclosings using the unsaturating disclosing procedure.

Disclosing with fluorescein also requires control of disclosing pH. Fluorescein fluoresces better at a lower pH and is optimal for tooth safety and stable fluorescence at pH 5.5. To control pH, the fluorescein is dosed in a glycerin base followed by a series of phosphate rinses to remove excess pooling of fluorescein and temporarily buffer plaque pH at 5.5.

Analysis of Images

Captured images are classified with Optimas® macros. The image pixels are classified using the least squared distance model summarized in the Appendix. The results of each analysis are written to an ascii text file and include subject ID, visit ID, analysis date, number of pixels of teeth, number of pixels of gingival plaque, number of pixels of plaque on teeth, percent plaque on teeth.

Figure 6 is an actual image, and figure 7 shows a generated classification image using the plaque-imaging system.

To test the reproducibility of the plaque analysis system, 6 volunteers refrained from oral hygiene for 12 h prior to having their plaque measured

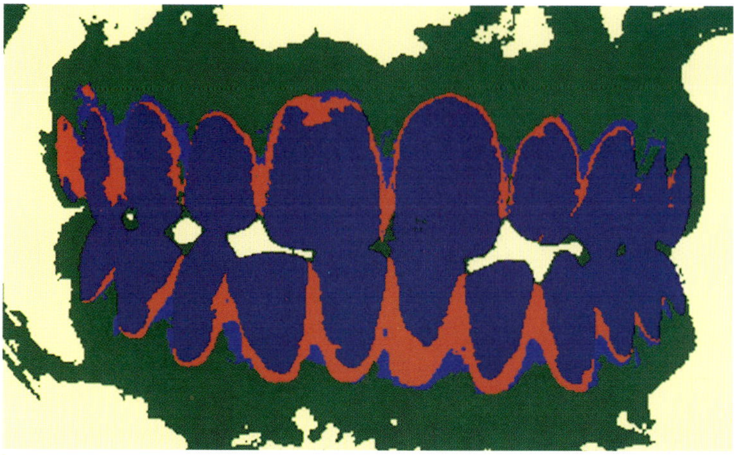

Fig. 7. Classification.

Table 2. Reproducibility Data

Measurement	Subject 1	Subject 2	Subject 3	Subject 4	Subject 5	Subject 6
1	30.8	21.7	29.2	6.62	15.2	21.6
2	31.4	22.5	29.2	5.83	14.9	23.8
3	33.3	22.2	30.8	6.22	14.9	21.0
Average	31.8	22.1	29.7	6.22	15.0	22.1
RSD	4.02	1.68	3.04	6.35	1.15	6.37

via digital plaque imaging. Each volunteer's plaque level was measured 3 consecutive times with redisclosing of their plaque between measurements. The average relative standard deviation of the measurements across the 6 volunteers was 3.77% indicating the repeatability of the measurement is good. The data are shown in table 2.

Application of Digital Plaque Image Analysis in a Crossover Test Evaluating 2 Commercial Dentifrices

The purpose of this test was to evaluate the relative plaque growth inhibition of Crest plus Gum Care compared to Crest Regular using digital plaque image analysis (DPIA) as the plaque-grading technique in a 10-subject product-crossover design.

Crest plus Gum Care provides clinically significant reductions in gingivitis and plaque [10, 11]. The active system, stabilized stannous fluoride, is a good inhibitor of ex vivo plaque glycolysis and regrowth. The mechanism of action is believed to be the inhibition of carbohydrate metabolism enzymes by stannous [12]. The clinical reductions in gingivitis and plaque are robust and are a good positive control for providing reductions in plaque level.

Materials and Methods

Ten volunteers refrained from oral hygiene for 12 h prior to measuring morning plaque levels using the DPIA technique. Prior to imaging plaque levels, a subject's plaque was disclosed with fluorescein and buffered with pH 5.5 phosphate buffer rinses.

Each subject's facial plaque was then digitally imaged within 60 s of completing the disclosing procedure.

Subjects brushed their entire dentition with 1.5 g of the designated test product (either Crest plus Gum Care or Crest Regular) for 2 min. After brushing, the subject's remaining plaque was redisclosed and area coverage measured with DPIA. This measurement serves as the baseline plaque level for regrowth.

Subjects used the test product two more times over the next 24 h: once after lunch, and once after dinner. For the final two brushings, the subjects brushed their lingual surfaces for 30 s and swished the developed slurry to the facial surfaces for 30 s. This technique allows a true evaluation of the chemotherapeutic efficacy of the agents as it accounts for in vivo brushing dilution and treatment without physically disrupting the facial surface plaque. No other oral hygiene was permitted for the overnight period.

Finally, each subject's plaque level was measured the next morning using the DPIA technique.

The procedure was repeated for both test products with half the subjects starting with Crest plus Gum Care and half starting with Crest Regular. There was a 4-day washout period between treatments.

All data were analyzed using ANOVA with subject and treatment as the main effects.

Results

Plaque Cleaning. Plaque cleaning is defined as the percent reduction in plaque level associated with the initial 2-min brushing. In terms of treatment, there were no significant differences in cleaning between Crest and Gum Care and Crest Regular as determined by contrast ANOVA with subject and treatment as the main effects. The results are summarized in table 3.

Post Brushing Plaque Levels. Plaque levels after the initial brushing serve as the baseline for evaluating the regrowth inhibition of the dentifrices. The

Table 3. Cleaning efficacy

Treatment	Reduction, %	2-tail p value vs. CR
Crest plus Gum Care	50.7	0.3233
Crest Regular	45.1	–

Table 4. Post-brushing plaque levels

Treatment	Coverage, %	2-tail p value vs. CR
Crest plus Gum Care	11.9	0.4459
Crest Regular	11.0	–

Table 5. Plaque regrowth inhibition

Treatment	Inhibition, %	2-tail p value vs. CR
Crest plus Gum Care	36.8	0.0015
Crest Regular	–12.9	–

post-brushing plaque levels are summarized in table 4. There were no differences in plaque level after brushing, thus verifying the balance between treatments for evaluating the regrowth inhibition of the treatments.

Plaque Regrowth Inhibition. The plaque regrowth inhibition is defined as the percent reduction in plaque level between the initial plaque level prior to whole mouth brushing and the plaque level the next morning after 3 treatments. In terms of treatment, Crest plus Gum Care significantly inhibited plaque regrowth better than Crest Regular (ANOVA). The results are summarized in table 5.

Plaque Growth. Plaque growth is defined as the absolute increase in plaque coverage from the initial post-brushing to the next morning. In terms of treatment effect, Crest plus Gum Care had a significantly lower amount of plaque regrowth. The results are summarized in table 6.

Discussion

The combination of the DPIA plaque area measurement method and the technique of brushing lingual surfaces and swishing the developed slurry

Table 6. Plaque growth

Treatment	Coverage increase, %	2-tail p value vs. CR
Crest plus Gum Care	2.85	0.0036
Crest Regular	14.0	–

to the facial surfaces is an excellent method for evaluating the chemotherapeutic plaque regrowth inhibition of dentifrice formulations. The method easily demonstrated the ability to measure plaque differences with a relatively small number of subjects in a crossover design. The technique allows in vivo dilution of the dentifrice to the correct amount as well as the critical interactions with saliva. By only brushing the lingual surfaces, the facial surface plaque is left physically undisturbed and the confounding effects of mechanical toothbrushing are eliminated from the plaque growth assessment. DPIA provides a precise measurement of plaque area on the facial surfaces.

Conclusions

DPIA is an excellent tool for measuring plaque levels in vivo. The method exhibits good reproducibility (RSD 3.77%) and can easily measure the plaque regrowth effects of known therapeutic plaque agents such as stannous. DPIA eliminates bias and reduces variability over traditional subjective plaque-grading techniques leading to higher quality data and more reliable clinical studies with fewer subjects and cost.

Appendix

Least Squared Distance Calculations

The notation used to descibe the method is as follows: R, G, B = Intensity value for red, green and blue for each pixel (0–255 scale); $\mathbf{x} = 1 \times 3$ matrix of red, green and blue values of pixel x; t = subscript denoting class (i.e. plaque, gums, etc.); $\mathbf{m}_t = 1 \times 3$ matrix containing mean RGB values of class t; $\mathbf{S}_t$ = RGB covariance matrix of class t; $|\mathbf{S}_t|$ = determinant of covariance matrix.

The mean RGB colors contained in $\mathbf{m}_t$ and the covariance matrix $\mathbf{S}_t$ for each class is calculated from sample pixels from representative images. The overnight plaque of 10 subjects was disclosed and digitally photographed under UV light. These images were sampled for pixels in each of the 5 classes. 150 pixels were sampled from each class across 5 classes and 10 subjects for a total of 7,500 pixels used to define means and variances of each of the classes.

The covariance matrix $\mathbf{S}_t$ for class t is:

$$\mathbf{S}_t = \begin{array}{c|ccc|} & \mathbf{R} & \mathbf{G} & \mathbf{B} \\ \mathbf{R} & \text{Cov}(R, R) & \text{Cov}(R, G) & \text{Cov}(R, B) \\ \mathbf{G} & \text{Cov}(R, G) & \text{Cov}(G, G) & \text{Cov}(B, G) \\ \mathbf{B} & \text{Cov}(R, B) & \text{Cov}(B, G) & \text{Cov}(B, B) \end{array}$$

$$\text{Cov}(\mathbf{X}, \mathbf{Y}) = 1/n \cdot \Sigma (\mathbf{X}_i - u_y)(\mathbf{Y}_i - u_y)$$

where: $\mathbf{X}_i$ and $\mathbf{Y}_i$ represent the i-th red, green or blue value in class t, and u_x and u_y are the mean red, green or blue value of class t.

The inverse matrix ($\mathbf{S}_t^{-1}$) is defined such that $\mathbf{S}_t^{-1} \cdot \mathbf{S}_t$ is the identity matrix:

$$\begin{array}{c|ccc|} & \mathbf{R} & \mathbf{G} & \mathbf{B} \\ \mathbf{R} & 1 & 0 & 0 \\ \mathbf{G} & 0 & 1 & 0 \\ \mathbf{B} & 0 & 0 & 1 \end{array}$$

The generalized squared distance from pixel $\mathbf{x}$ to class t is given by the following equation:

$$D_t^2(\mathbf{x}) = (\mathbf{x} - \mathbf{m}_t)' \cdot \mathbf{S}_t^{-1} \cdot (\mathbf{x} - \mathbf{m}_t) + \log |\mathbf{S}_t| .$$

The pixel is then classified into the class where the distance is at a minimum. The probability of pixel $\mathbf{x}$ belonging to class t is then given by:

$$p(^x \mid t) = e_t^{-.5D(x)} / \Sigma e_i^{-.5D_i(x)}.$$

References

1 Breuer MM, Cosgrove RS: The relationship between gingivitis and plaque levels. J Periodontol 1989;60:172–175.

2 Loe H: The gingival index, the plaque index and the retention index systems. J Periodontol 1967; 38:610–616.

3 Fischman SL: Current status of indices of plaque. J Clin Periodontol 1986;13:371–374.

4 Ainamo J, Etemadzadeh H, Kallio P: Comparibility and discriminating power of four plaque quantifications. J Clin Periodontol 1993;20:244–249.

5 Soder PO, Jin LJ, Soder B: Computerized planimetric method for clinical plaque measurement. Scand J Dent Res 1993;101:21–25.

6 Poulsen S, Holm-Pedersen P, Kelstrup J: Comparison of different measurements of development of plaque and gingivitis in man. Scand J Dent Res 1979;87:178–183.

7 Mander CI, Mainwarning PJ: Assessment of the validity of two plaque indices. Community Dent Oral Epidemiol 1980;8:139–141.

8 Quirynen M, Deheyser C, van Steenberghe D: Discriminating power of five plaque indices. J Periodentol 1991;62:100–105.

9 MacGregor IDM: Comparison of the Silness-Loe (1964) index with gravimetric measurement of dental plaque. Clin Prev Dent 1987;9:9–12.

10 Gillings B: Recent developments in dental plaque disclosants. Aust Dent J 1977;22:260–266.
11 Lang N: A fluorescent plaque disclosing agent. J Periodont Res 1972;7:59–67.
12 Marks RG, Magnusson I, Taylor M, Clouser B, Maruniak J, Clark WB: Evaluation of reliability and reproducibility of dental indices. J Clin Periodontol 1993;20:54–58.
13 Perlich MA, Bacca LA, Bollmer BW, Lanzalaco AC, McClanahan SF, Sewak LK, Beiswanger BB, Eichold WA, Hull JR, Jackson RD: The clinical effect of a stabilized stannous fluoride dentifrice on plaque formation, gingivitis, and gingival bleeding: A six month study. J Clin Dent 1995;6(special issue):54–58.
14 Beiswanger BB: The clinical effect of dentifrices containing stabilized stannous fluoride on plaque formation and gingivitis – A six month study with ad libitum brushing. J Clin Dent 1995;6(special issue):46–53.
15 White DJ: A new plaque glycolysis and regrowth method (PGRM) for the in vivo determination of anti-microbial dentifrice/rinse efficacy towards the inhibition of plaque growth and metabolism: Method development, validation and initial activity screens. J Clin Dent 1995;6(special issue):59–70.

Paul A. Sagel, Procter & Gamble Company, Health Care Research Center,
PO Box 8006, Mason, OH 45040-8006 (USA)
Tel. +1 513 622 2688, Fax +1 513 622 3508, E-Mail sagel.pa@pg.com

Faller RV (ed): Assessment of Oral Health.
Monogr Oral Sci. Basel, Karger, 2000, vol 17, pp 144–162

Application of Quantitative Light-Induced Fluorescence for Assessing Early Caries Lesions

M.H. van der Veen[a, b], *E. de Josselin de Jong*[b]

[a] ACTA, Department of Cariology, Endodontology and Pedodontology, and
[b] Inspektor Research Systems b.v., Amsterdam, The Netherlands

Abstract

Quantitative light induced fluorescence (QLF) is a nondestructive diagnostic method for the longitudinal assessment of early caries lesions in time. When a tooth becomes carious the fluorescence radiance at the location of the caries lesion decreases. The fluorescence image of enamel with incipient lesions can be digitized and then the fluorescence loss in the lesion can be quantified in comparison to the fluorescence radiance level of sound enamel. Changes in fluorescence radiance and lesion area can be followed in time to measure lesion development. The amount of fluorescence radiance loss is related to the mineral loss in the lesion. The technique can be used in vitro, in situ and in vivo to monitor mineral changes in lesions. Applications of QLF are found in the testing of products designed to inhibit demineralization and promote remineralization of caries. The method has been successfully applied to smooth surfaces as well as occlusal surfaces, but application on approximal lesions is not yet possible.

Need for Noninvasive Quantitative Detection Methods in Dentistry

First of all the dentist uses his or her eyes when judging teeth for the absence or presence of caries. The appearance of detected caries lesions is judged for color (white or brown), lesion reflectance (shiny or dull) and surface texture (rough or smooth). Based on the lesion appearance and caries incidence history of the patient, the dentist will decide on a treatment plan.

Over the past decades the emphasis in dentistry has shifted from restorative treatment towards prevention of new caries progression and arrest or demineralization of existing caries. It is believed that incipient lesions can be remineralized more effectively than more advanced lesions. Therefore it is important to detect caries lesions when they are still incipient and monitor lesion development to check the effectiveness of preventive treatment until complete remineralization is achieved.

An incipient lesion viewed directly on a smooth surface appears whiter than the surrounding enamel under normal white light illumination. Therefore it is called a white spot lesion. Lesions in fissures or on approximal surfaces are viewed directly as well as indirectly, e.g. by transillumination, where they appear as a dark shadow on the surface viewed.

The methods available for caries detection are already quite good at finding incipient lesions. With the exception of approximal surfaces the visual detection system is hard to beat by instrumental methods designed to measure presence or absence of caries only. Research for new caries diagnostic methods should aim at complementing the visual observation [1].

One of these additions is quantification of lesions after detection. Quantification of lesion parameters, e.g. lesion area, depth and mineral loss, may lead to a better evaluation of such lesions. Diagnosis may become more precise and may become a longitudinal process in which lesion changes over time are evaluated.

Quantitative light-induced fluorescence (QLF) is a diagnostic technique that uses the natural fluorescence of teeth to discriminate between caries and sound enamel and to give a measure of lesion severity. The fluorescence radiance of a carious lesion viewed with QLF is lower than that of sound enamel. To date, an observed relationship between mineral loss and fluorescence radiance [2–5] has been accepted. The loss in fluorescence radiance can be followed longitudinally to monitor mineral changes in a lesion [6]. The observation of longitudinal mineral changes will enable us to determine the effect of advice and treatment tailored to inhibit demineralization and promote remineralization of caries lesions.

Development of QLF

Bjelkhagen and Sundström [7], Bjelkhagen et al. [8] and Sundström et al. [9] first described the use of laser autofluorescence (LAF) for the qualitative assessment of mineral loss. These studies demonstrated in vivo enhancement of contrast between incipient lesions and sound enamel examined using laser fluorescence compared with normal white light. Using white light illumination, lesions may be obscured by reflections from the surrounding tooth surface

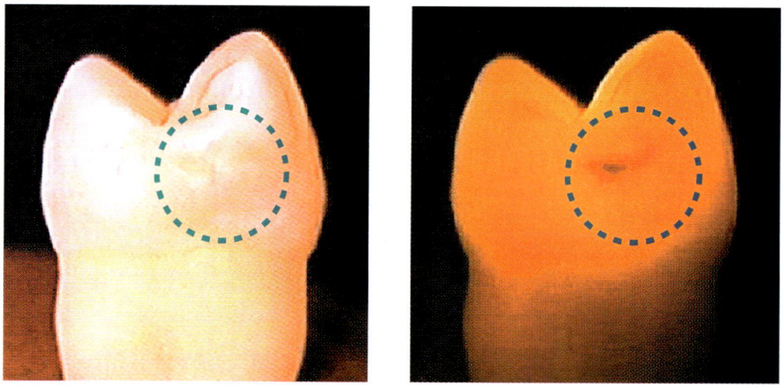

Fig. 1. Comparison of a white light image of a premolar tooth compared with a laser fluorescence image. The circle highlights the position of the incipient carious lesion. Note the reflections on the white light image which obscure the lesion. From de Josselin de Jong et al. [15].

whereas with LAF, the lesion can be observed clearly (fig. 1). The LAF method used a powerful Argon laser emitting blue light with $\lambda = 488$ nm (at 50 mW continuous wave, corresponding to ~ 20 mW/cm^2 at the tooth surface) to illuminate the teeth. A yellow cutoff filter ($\lambda \geq 520$ nm), filtering out all reflected and back scattered light, was placed in front of the eye in order to view the lesion. In 1992 a quantitative LAF system for determination of mineral loss was described [2]. This method was further developed as an intra-oral laser fluorescence system [10] to assess the baseline mineral content and longitudinal change in the mineral content of early enamel lesions in vivo.

To date a laboratory system and a portable intra-oral camera for QLF measurements are available [11–13]. In these systems the laser was replaced by an arc lamp in combination with a bandpass filter to provide illumination of the teeth with blue-violet light.

Optical Principles of QLF Observation of White Spot Lesions

QLF uses the natural fluorescence of the teeth. There is no need for application of dyes or other enhancers. With QLF the observer looks at a dark lesion, where in normal daylight without special filters one would see a white spot in a 'white' surrounding. A lesion viewed with light-induced fluorescence is not obscured by reflections that obstruct the image of a lesion when viewed under normal white light conditions. The dark appearance of a white spot lesion viewed with the fluorescence technique can be explained by the changes in scattering properties occurring in a lesion [14, 15].

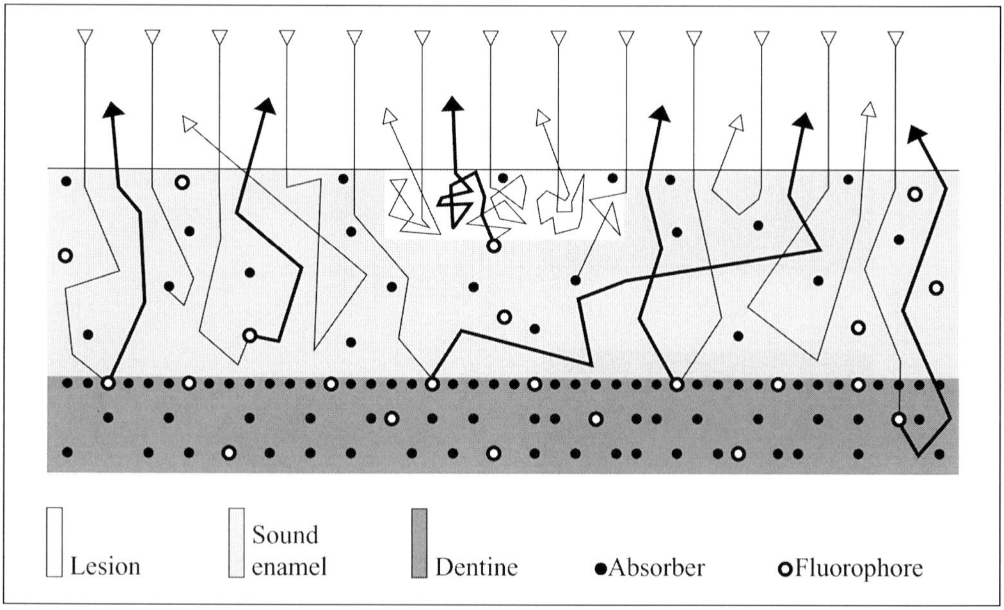

Fig. 2. A schematic overview of the scattering, absorption and fluorescence in sound and carious enamel with sound dentine underneath. The penetration depth of light in the lesion is smaller than in sound enamel. Photons entering carious enamel are highly scattered. Most light entering the lesion is volume reflected from the lesion and the chance of photon absorption and fluorescence is small. Light entering the lesion does not reach the dentin. Light entering sound enamel is scattered about a factor of 10 less than in carious enamel. Photons travel further in sound enamel and along their path may be absorbed by a fluorophore leading to excitation of fluorescent photons. Light entering sound enamel may reach the DEJ and dentine where the chance of absorption by a fluorophore is a magnitude higher. Many more fluorescence photons are emitted from the sound enamel than from the lesion. To simplify the scheme it is assumed that all fluorescent photons are remitted towards the enamel surface. In reality all directions of fluorescent photon remittance from the fluorophore are equally likely.

The scattering coefficient of a white spot lesion is a factor 5 to 10 higher than that of the surrounding sound enamel [16]. In a white spot lesion the incident light is scattered more often than in sound enamel. This is caused by the disintegration of the crystalline structure resulting in more internal reflection sites. Increased scattering implies that the 'mean free path of photon transport' inside a lesion is shorter than in sound enamel. The chance for a photon to be absorbed and fluorescence remitted is therefore higher in the sound enamel than in the white spot and we assume that more fluorescent light is remitted from the sound enamel than from the lesion.

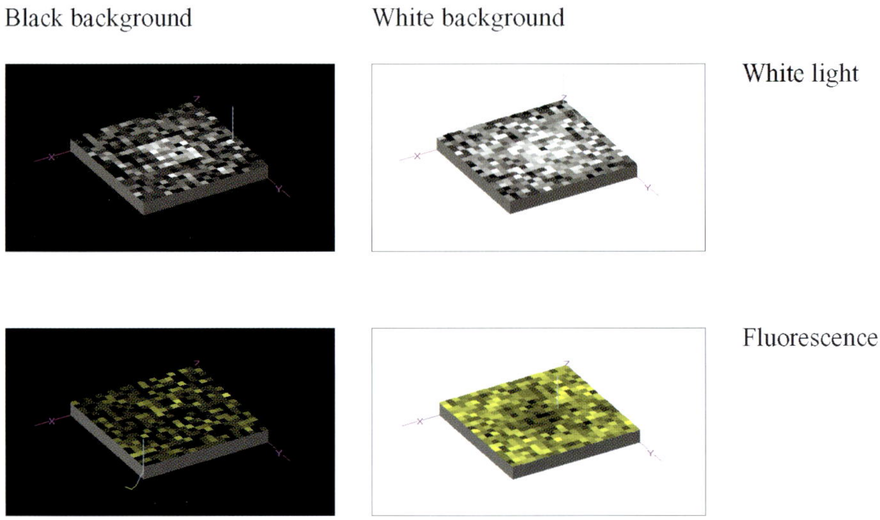

Fig. 3. Images from the model to simulate how mineral loss may be observed against black and white backgrounds using white light and the fluorescence technique. Note the similarity between these images and those in figure 4. From de Josselin de Jong et al. [15].

The effect of scattering on the appearance of a white spot lesion viewed with light-induced fluorescence is enhanced by the highly fluorescing nature of dentine and even more so the dentin-enamel junction (DEJ). Light entering the white spot does not reach the DEJ or dentine but is back scattered and for a minor part remitted as fluorescence light from the lesion. Light entering the sound enamel can reach the DEJ or dentine where it is more likely to be remitted as fluorescence. As a result we see a dark lesion surrounded by highly luminescent sound enamel (fig. 2).

This theoretical scattering model as an explanation of light-induced fluorescence was tested using Monte Carlo simulation [15]. The scattering coefficient of sound enamel was set to 10/mm and that of the white spot was set to 250/mm. The outcome of the Monte Carlo simulation (fig. 3) was then compared to a simple experiment where images of an enamel slab with a white spot were captured using light-induced fluorescence and white light scattering. To represent the presence or absence of dentine and DEJ, the enamel slab was placed on either a bright fluorescent white background or a nonfluorescent black background, respectively (fig. 4). The Monte Carlo simulation and the in vitro experiment had the same results: (1) a lesion observed in white light on a white background appears whiter than the surrounding 'white' enamel,

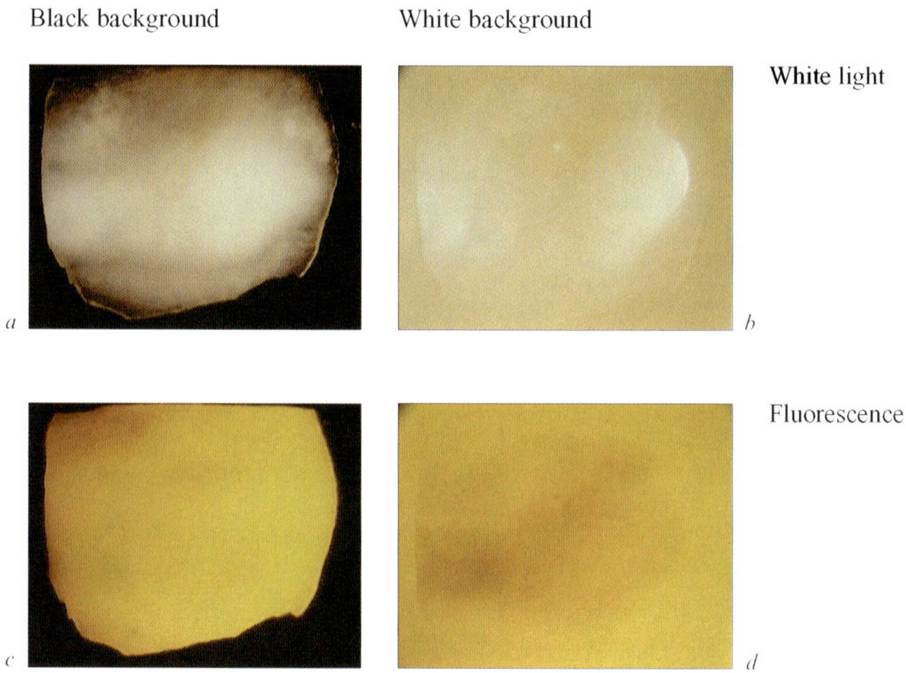

Fig. 4. Comparison of images of a tooth slice with a natural incipient lesion cut from a premolar tooth. Images have been captured with black and white backgrounds using white light and the fluorescence technique. *b, d* The clinical situation for smooth surface lesions. From de Josselin de Jong et al. [15].

contrast between the lesion and sound enamel is low; (2) a lesion observed in white light on a dark background appears as a white spot surrounded by dark sound enamel, contrast is high; (3) a lesion observed with light-induced fluorescence on a white background appears dark compared to highly luminescent surrounding enamel, contrast is high, and (4) a lesion observed with light-induced fluorescence on a black background appears dark and not distinguishable from the surrounding sound enamel.

Points 1 and 3 describe the normal situation of a tooth with dentine present under the enamel viewed in white light or with light-induced fluorescence, respectively. Although fluorescence and white light appearance of a lesion are mainly due to the scattering phenomenon in tooth tissue, the visual effects behave very differently.

The results show that the Monte Carlo simulation adequately simulates white spots in enamel and it may be concluded that scattering and absorption are the main factors accounting for the fluorescence effect. The presence of the DEJ or dentine underneath the enamel is needed to provide good fluorescence contrast between the lesion and the sound enamel.

The relationship found between fluorescence radiance loss and mineral loss from a lesion [2, 4, 5, 11] and mineral gain [12, 17, 18] becomes evident knowing that there is a strong correlation between mineral loss in a lesion and scattering coefficient [19].

Application of QLF

QLF is an optical technique to assess early caries lesions in enamel. QLF is suitable to follow enamel de- and remineralizations longitudinally in a clinical situation as well as in the laboratory. This gives QLF a great potential for in vitro and in vivo product testing, but also as a supporting method to follow the effect of preventive treatment of patients in a dental office.

So far QLF has proven successful in a number of in vitro re- and demineralization studies and several clinical studies on remineralization of, e.g. white-spot lesions after debracketing of orthodontic patients [20]. Some preliminary data of a larger clinical trial were presented recently [21–23].

The first studies with QLF were designed to validate QLF against accepted laboratory techniques suited to measure mineral loss and/or lesion depth. A correlation as high as $r = 0.97$ was found with mineral loss [2, 4, 5, 11].

The method was used in vitro to test the effect of different protocols on lesion inhibition and remineralization [12, 17, 24]. Normally in such studies only baseline and end readings of mineral loss or hardness can be measured, but QLF offers the ability to measure changes in fluorescence loss at time intervals during the study after which the remineralization protocol can be continued. This gives important information on the initial remineralization speed of a product and when remineralization starts to slow down.

QLF has also found its use for longitudinal monitoring of enamel remineralization in in situ studies [18]. In this study fluorescence was regained up to 80–100% of the sound enamel fluorescence level. The fluorescence gain correlated ($r = 0.76$) with the mineral gain found with transverse microradiography (TMR).

A small-sized clinical trial with QLF was performed on 7 orthodontic patients after debracketing [20] to validate QLF for longitudinal measurements of caries in vivo. Orthodontic patients are highly susceptible to caries [25]. The area around the brackets is difficult to clean and hence it is prone to caries attack. Lesions are formed rapidly and are very active. The lesions developed around the brackets can be remineralized when proper oral hygiene is provided [26]. This makes orthodontic patients very suitable for clinical trials with QLF. To study the effect of different treatment regimes the lesion severity needs to be followed in time. With QLF we get a standardized measure of the lesion area and the loss of fluorescence radiance in that lesion. The increase or decrease of those measures shows us the effect of the treatment protocol. The best representation of lesion progression or regression is given by the longitudinal changes in ΔQ, where ΔQ is defined as the fluorescence loss integrated over the lesion area ($\% \cdot mm^2$). ΔQ is comparable to the amount of mineral loss measured with longitudinal microradiography [27]. The QLF study by Al-Khateeb et al. [20] showed partial regression of the lesions over a 1-year period. An example of a lesion analyzed with QLF directly after debracketing and followed for 9 months during remineralization treatment is given in figure 5. The authors conclude that QLF is suitable for longitudinal monitoring of caries in vivo and that QLF is useful for the evaluation of preventive measures in caries-prone persons.

A 6-month clinical trial on caries-active teenagers was presented by Tranaeus et al. [28]. In this study repeated treatment with fluoride varnish was compared to frequent professional tooth cleaning as a means to promote demineralization. Thirty teenagers with 2 white spot lesions each were assigned to either the fluoride varnish group or the tooth-cleaning group. The results showed a $6.8 \pm 16.6\%$ increase in fluorescence and a $14.2 \pm 30.2\%$ decrease in lesion area for the fluoride varnish treatment ($p < 0.05$) and corresponding changes of 11.2 ± 20.1 and $21.4 \pm 51.8\%$ for the professional tooth cleaning group (not significant). In high-risk patients fluoride varnish treatment had a favorable effect over professional tooth cleaning after 6 months.

Preliminary results from a larger clinical trial on 150 children with mixed dentition showed the repeatability of QLF for the detection of caries [21] and quantification of such caries [22]. QLF detected 9.5 times more demineralized surfaces than the full-mouth clinical examinations [29]. Eight-month longitudinal data from a subset of 14 panelists showed lesion regression for 2 months ($p < 0.05$) and no significant changes afterwards [23]. A pilot study was conducted before the start of the clinical trial to validate QLF for quantification of lesions in the deciduous dentition [30]. Results showed that lesions of same depth were easier to detect on deciduous teeth than on permanent teeth and the correlation with TMR was strongest for the lesions in deciduous enamel. Findings from this study were supported by a Monte Carlo simulation that studied the effect of differences in scattering coefficient of sound enamel on the appearance of a lesion with QLF [31]. In figure 6 graphs showing the influence of the sound enamel scattering coefficient on the fluorescence or white light imaging of lesions are presented.

Smooth Surface Lesions

QLF is best suited for longitudinal diagnoses of early enamel lesions on directly accessible smooth surfaces. Analysis of detected lesions is not hindered

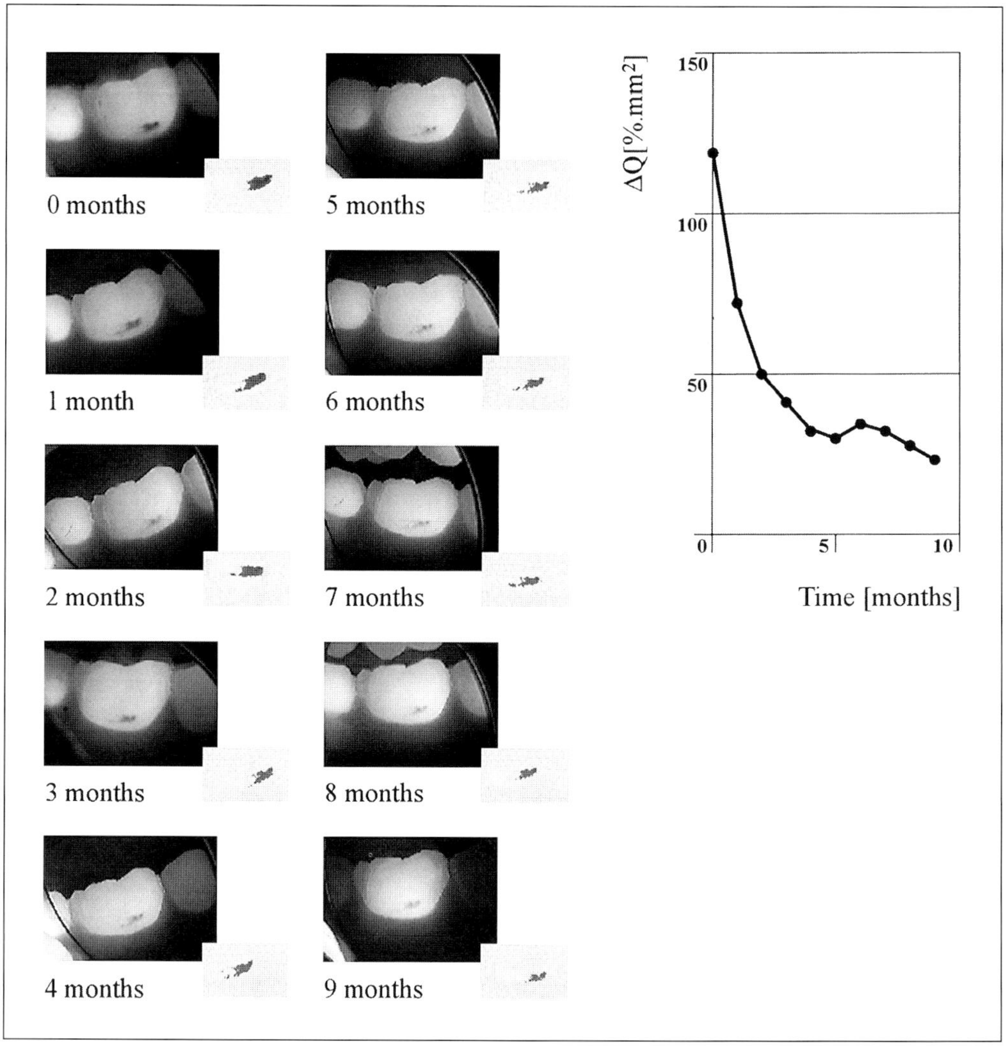

Fig. 5. Longitudinal images of a permanent first molar after debracketing. Images of the tooth were captured monthly for 9 months. The insets show the analyzed lesion area. Pixels with a fluorescence radiance level of $<95\%$ compared to sound enamel were considered caries and are shown in gray. Darker gray stands for more fluorescence loss. The graph shows the change in ΔQ defined as fluorescence radiance loss (%) $\times$ lesion area (mm^2) over the 9-month period. The lesion shows signs of remineralization as can be seen on the QLF images and, more clearly, in the graph. Courtesy of S. Al-Khateeb.

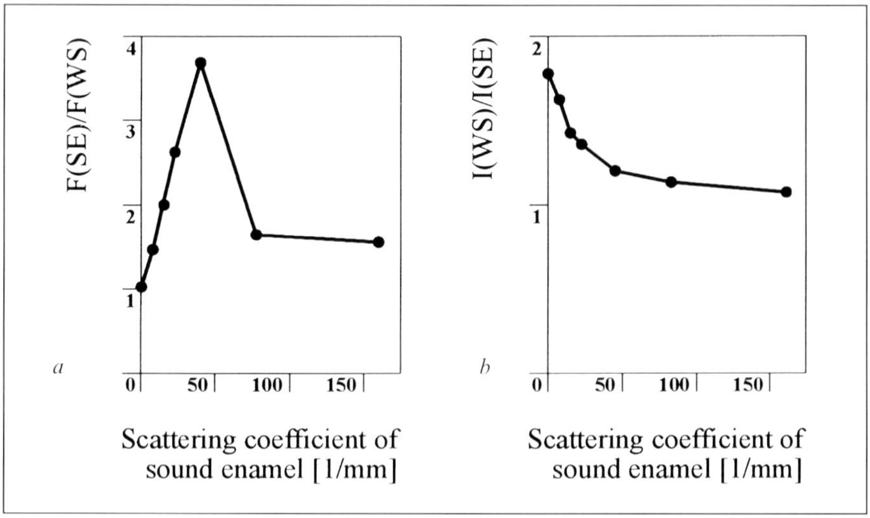

Fig. 6. The relationship between lesion visibility and the sound enamel scattering coefficient used in Monte Carlo simulations of fluorescence (*a*) or white light scattering (*b*) images of a sound enamel slab with a white spot lesion. Lesion visibility for the fluorescence simulations is expressed as the number of fluorescent photons remitted from the sound enamel per unit area F(SE) divided by the number of fluorescent photons remitted from the lesion per unit area F(WS). Lesion visibility for the white light scattering simulations is expressed as the number of backscattered photons from the white spot per unit area I(WS) divided by number of backscattered photons from the sound enamel per unit area I(SE). Due to edge losses for low sound enamel scattering coefficients the fluorescence remitted from sound enamel is lowered resulting in less contrast between the lesion and sound enamel, whereas for white light scattering the contrast is enhanced.

by the lesions being located in pits or fissures below the surface or even on a different surface as is the case with approximal lesions. Examples of in vitro smooth surface applications of QLF are described by Sundström et al. [32], Hall et al. [33], Ando et al. [5] and Al-Khateeb et al. [17]. A model for in situ application of QLF for product testing was introduced by Al-Khateeb et al. [18]. Clinical application of QLF on smooth surfaces to follow lesion development in orthodontic patients after debracketing was presented by Al-Khateeb et al. [20]. Tranaeus et al. [28] performed a study involving the buccal surfaces of two teeth only to study different treatments in a group of caries-prone teenagers.

Pits and Fissures

Most studies of lesions in pits and fissures have been aiming at detection rather than longitudinal follow-up of lesions [34–36]. In these studies QLF

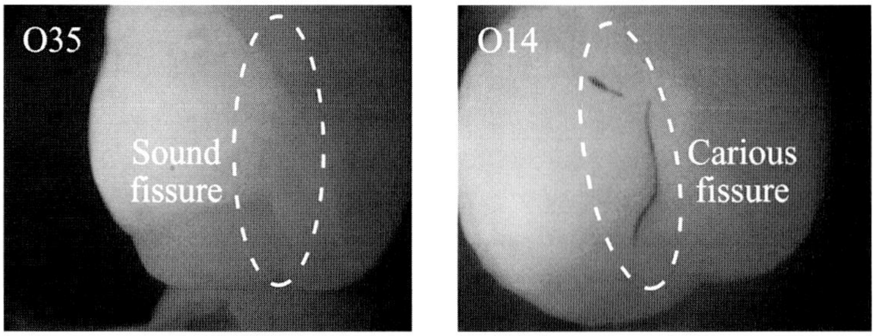

a *b*

Fig. 7. Images of the occlusal surfaces of two permanent premolars with sound fissures (*a*) and an incipient fissure lesion (*b*). The fissure areas are encircled.

was compared to dye-enhanced laser fluorescence (DELF) and visual examination for the detection of lesions. Lesion presence or absence was determined with histology, confocal laser scanning microscopy and TMR. Results indicated that DELF gives a higher sensitivity and similar specificity than QLF or visual examination. Visual examination is as good as QLF when the dentist is instructed to look at early signs of caries, i.e. color changes. The ability of QLF to quantify the lesion area and fluorescence loss was not used in these studies.

Tranaeus et al. [37] compared QLF for detection and quantification of occlusal caries with other methods such as visual inspection, bitewing radiography and electrical conductance measurements. The level of fluorescence loss observed was used to decide whether caries had progressed into dentine. A cutoff level of 20% fluorescence radiance loss was chosen. QLF showed sensitivity and specificity values of 0.71 and 0.73, respectively, which were lower than those for electrical conductance measurements (0.93 and 0.98). These are promising results but further development of QLF for use on occlusal surfaces is needed. A different illumination and camera configuration, of illumination and observation of the fissure under the same angle may help [35, 36].

To date only one clinical trial has longitudinally monitored changes in lesions on all surfaces including lesions located in pits and fissures [23]. Preliminary data showing a decrease in lesion size and fluorescence loss were given for a subset of subjects, but specific data on the lesions in pits and fissures are not yet available. Examples of an occlusal surface with sound fissures and an occlusal surface with incipient fissure lesion are given in figure 7.

Approximal Lesions

QLF in its present state is not suitable for use on approximal lesions. The geometry of incident light beam and camera makes it virtually impossible to detect approximal lesions at an early stage. Tooth shape and the location of approximal lesions under the contact point make it hard to get light at the lesion site and to view from almost the same direction. When an approximal lesion is observed from an adjacent tooth surface we look at a cross-section of the lesion or the lesion depth which is extremely small in comparison to the lesion surface. Since there is no dentine below the enamel when an approximal surface is viewed from buccal, lingual or occlusal surface the contrast between the lesion and the surrounding enamel is very low. Only when the dentine becomes carious may we expect to see something.

Eggertsson et al. [38] have tried to use laser fluorescence for the detection of approximal lesions in an attempt to find an illumination and imaging geometry that would enhance lesion detection compared to visual examination. In vitro lesions with an average depth of 60 μm were placed in approximal geometry and examined visually, QLF, and DELF. Bitewing radiography was also tried but the lesions were not visible on the radiographs at all. All three techniques showed similar results for sensitivity and specificity. Lesions were detected by the illumination of the area below the contact point and viewing the area from almost the same direction, although the examiners were encouraged to use different light and viewing geometries. In the clinical situation the direct view of approximal lesions is obstructed by the gingiva. With this configuration, quantification is not possible because at most only part of the lesion can be observed.

When QLF is to be used for approximal caries also, illumination from below the contact area and observance of the area from the occlusal surface as is used in fiber-optic transillumination may be more effective.

Lesions Next to Restorative Materials

Several attempts have been made to use QLF for detection, quantification and longitudinal monitoring of secondary caries lesions. The best approaches so far were all looking at artificial lesions on the enamel surface adjacent to amalgam fillings [24, 39, 40] or tooth colored restorations [40, 41]. These studies all show the ability of QLF to detect lesions and quantify the fluorescence loss and lesion area. Examples of natural caries lesions adjacent to amalgam or composite resin restorations are given in figure 8. Whether the caries observed is true secondary caries or primary caries left when the restoration was placed is unknown.

Hall et al. [24] also made an attempt to follow lesion regression as a result of a pH-cycling procedure aimed at remineralization. On enamel specimens lesions were created in vitro in a small window next to an amalgam filling. The specimens were analyzed with QLF to determine initial fluorescence loss and this was compared to mineral loss found with TMR. The sections cut for

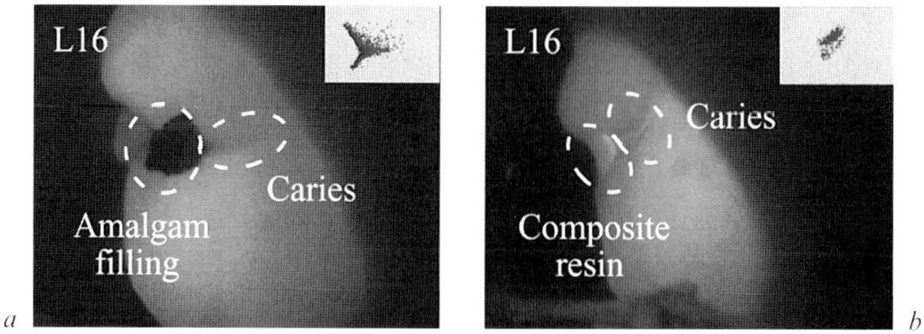

Fig. 8. Images of the lingual surfaces of two first permanent molars with caries (encircled) next to restorations. The occlusal surfaces were restored with amalgam (*a*) or composite resin (*b*). Amalgam does not display fluorescence and will be excluded as a lesion during analysis based on its dark color in comparison with both the sound enamel and the lesion (*a* inset). Composite resin may display lower, equal or more fluorescence than sound enamel depending on the filler material. To analyze the lesion next to the composite the border between composite resin and lesion needs to be determined and excluded from the analysis (*b* inset).

TMR and the remaining bulk specimens were both subjected to the same remineralization protocol. Fluorescence gain measured with QLF and mineral gain measured with TMR corresponded indicating that QLF is suitable for monitoring mineral changes in lesions next to restorations.

Quantification of Lesions with QLF

When a dentist has identified a caries lesion on a tooth surface, an image of the surface is captured. The lesion is marked on a screen to ensure analysis of only those areas determined as caries. The lesion is analyzed using a user-defined patch with borders placed on sound enamel surrounding the lesion. The sound fluorescence radiance values inside the patch are reconstructed through two-dimensional linear interpolation of sound enamel values on the patch borders [10]. The decrease in fluorescence is determined by calculating the percentage difference between actual and reconstructed fluorescence surface. In general an area with a fluorescence radiance drop of more than 5% is considered carious (figure 9).

For in vitro lesions, homogeneously formed and of fixed size, fluorescence radiance loss is used to follow lesion severity in time with QLF. In vivo lesions are inhomogeneous and the lesion area varies in time. Thus, not only the fluorescence radiance but also the lesion area must be monitored to follow lesion progression or regression. QLF measures fluorescence radiance loss (%)

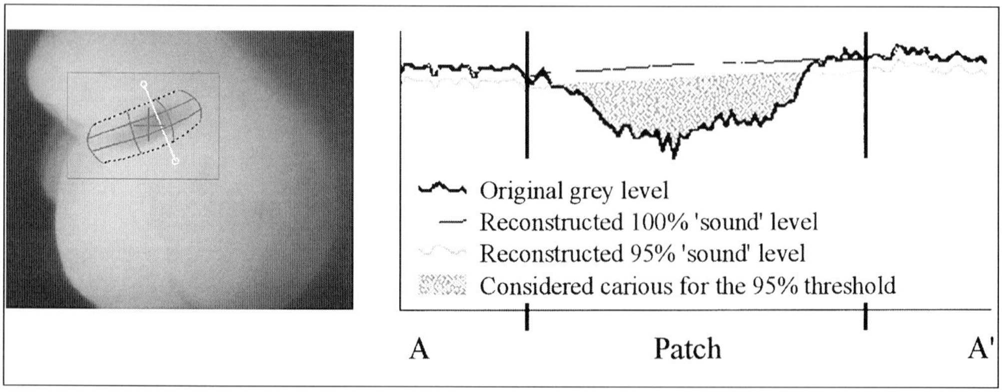

Fig. 9. The change in fluorescence radiance is measured with respect to the fluorescence radiance level of sound enamel in the same image. The line histogram along the line AA′ shows both the reconstructed sound fluorescence radiance levels and the actual fluorescence radiance levels. The pixels along the line AA′ across the analysis patch with a fluorescence radiance level <95% of the reconstructed sound enamel fluorescence radiance level are considered carious and are marked in gray.

and lesion size (mm^2) as well as ΔQ ($\% \cdot mm^2$) to describe lesion severity. ΔQ is defined as the fluorescence radiance loss integrated over the lesion area ($\% \cdot mm^2$). ΔQ is comparable to the total amount of mineral lost from the lesion as measured with longitudinal microradiography. For clinical studies ΔQ is the lesion parameter to be monitored in time [27].

Lesions in Pits or Fissures

For lesions in pits and fissures the tooth morphology causes an inhomogeneous fluorescence pattern with shadowing around the fissures. To ensure proper reconstruction of such areas the linear interpolation lines connecting two points on opposite patch borders can be curved to follow the shadowing on the tooth.

Lesions Adjacent to Restorations

Figure 8 displays the images of lingual surfaces of two permanent first molars with caries next to an amalgam restoration (fig. 8a) or composite resin (fig. 8b). Amalgam does not fluoresce and will be excluded during analysis based on its dark appearance in comparison with sound enamel and the lesion. The patch border crossing the amalgam is not used to reconstruct sound fluorescence radiance values within the patch. Areas with fluorescence radiance values of <20% of the reconstructed sound fluorescence radiance values are considered to be part of the amalgam restoration. Areas with fluorescence radiance values between 20 and 95% of the reconstructed sound fluorescence radiance values are considered carious.

Composite resin may display lower, equal or more fluorescence than sound enamel depending on the type and amount of filler material. Glass ionomer restorations always show brighter fluorescence than sound enamel. To analyze the lesion next to composite or glass ionomer restorations one of the patch borders needs to follow the border between the restoration and the lesion and that border, i.e. the restoration, must be excluded from the analysis.

Scaling Correction

The intra-oral QLF camera is a hand-held device and thus the distance between the tooth surface and camera sensor is never exactly the same. To provide some standardization of distance, tips on the head of the hand piece are used to hold the camera at a 'fixed' distance from the tooth. To correct for differences in scaling occurring as a result of the manual positioning, the QLF software uses a zoom factor.

For longitudinal measurements, markers on the contour of the surface are used to correct for differences in the distance between camera and tooth surface. Analysis patch and contour are grouped and copied to all longitudinal images of the same tooth surface. The contour is resized to fit the tooth surface in each of the images such that scaling factors are adjusted for. This way the analysis patch is always placed on the same location of the surface and the area inside the patch has always the same size.

Discussion

QLF is a technique intended to assist in caries diagnosis through quantification of lesion severity and longitudinal monitoring of lesion severity in time. Whether or not a dark spot on a tooth as observed with QLF is a lesion has to be decided based upon normal white light visual examination. Once a dark spot is determined as a caries lesion the lesion can be followed in time to determine lesion activity. Most QLF studies performed so far did not monitor caries longitudinally, but emphasized caries detection and quantification at one point in time. Based on one-time quantification of a lesion one cannot discriminate between active and inactive lesions.

Tranaeus et al. [37] used a lesion fluorescence loss level of 20% to diagnose dentinal caries. However, QLF was not designed to discriminate between lesions restricted to the enamel and lesions extending into the dentine. The fluorescence loss levels measured with a specific QLF camera are influenced by the system specifications [13] and for each camera the relation between fluorescence loss and mineral loss, lesion depth or dentinal involvement has to be calibrated.

With QLF it is possible to study single lesions on tooth surfaces to provide information about, e.g. treatment effects on occlusal lesions versus smooth surface lesions. Behavior of lesions with different lesion severity within one panellist to the same treatment may give information about the level of lesion severity above which remineralization is no longer feasible.

Changes in lesion area and fluorescence radiance loss together give a measure of the changes in lesion severity. In clinical studies of natural caries lesions the measure that should be followed over time is ΔQ ($\% \cdot mm^2$), which is defined as the lesion area (mm^2) multiplied by the mean change in fluorescence radiance (%). For in vitro studies where the lesion area is kept constant the mean change in fluorescence radiance should be followed in time.

Brown Spots, Surface Stains and Plaque

In general a brown spot viewed with light-induced fluorescence will appear dark, just like a white spot lesion. The absorption of light in the brown spot may enhance the fluorescence loss observed when the area was not discolored. Ferreira Zandoná et al. [36] found that discoloration of enamel was an indicator of enamel demineralization. White light visual examination will have to distinguish between brown stains located on or in the enamel. Longitudinal examinations are needed to determine the lesion activity.

Also plaque may obstruct a lesion. Plaque may appear dark, but can also be bright red fluorescent. Proper cleaning of the tooth surface is needed prior to QLF imaging and lesion analysis.

Discrimination between Fluorosis and Lesions

Fluorosis viewed with light-induced fluorescence gives a similar appearance as white spot lesions as a dark spot surrounded by bright fluorescent sound enamel [42]. This may lead to ill conclusions in detection of caries.

In general the location and pattern of fluorosis is different than from enamel caries (fig. 10). Also we assume that size and porosity of fluorosis do not change over time, whereas caries is a dynamic process. In cases where we are uncertain about our diagnosis of a white spot being fluorosis or caries it is recommended to follow the development over time. When we see change, caries is involved and treatment can be given and monitored accordingly.

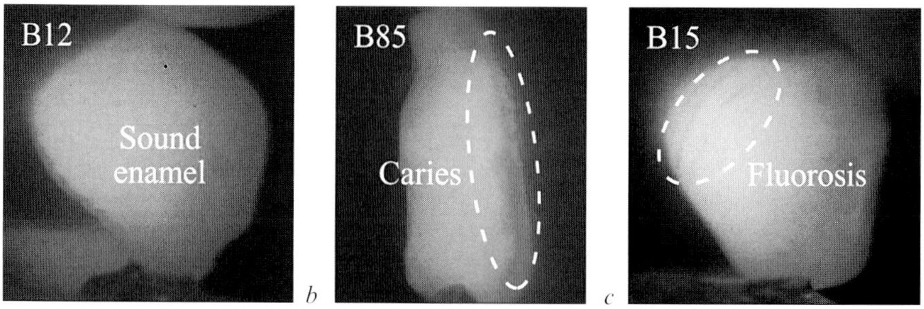

Fig. 10. a A sound buccal surface of a lateral tooth. *b* The buccal surface of a deciduous molar with cervical caries (encircled). *c* The buccal surface of a permanent premolar displaying very mild fluorosis (encircled). The caries lesion is irregularly shaped with no sharp boundaries. Fluorosis is recognized by the regular pattern and sharp boundaries.

Conclusions

QLF is a suitable tool for monitoring mineral changes in incipient enamel lesions. QLF can be used in vitro, in situ and in vivo. The method is equally suited for deciduous and permanent dentition thus allowing the method to be used for caries monitoring in children as well as adults.

Clinical use of QLF is not restricted to smooth surfaces alone but may include occlusal surfaces. QLF for the application on approximal surfaces needs further development.

References

1 ten Bosch JJ: General aspects of optical methods in dentistry. Adv Dent Res 1987;1:5–7.
2 Hafström-Björkman U, Sundström F, de Josselin de Jong E, Oliveby A, Angmar-Månsson B: Comparison of laser fluorescence and longitudinal microradiography for quantitative assessment of in vitro enamel caries. Caries Res 1992;26:241–247.
3 Emami Z, de Josselin de Jong E, Sundström F, Angmar-Månsson B: Quantification of mineral loss in initial caries on natural enamel surfaces with laser fluorescence and longitudinal microradiography (abstract 36). Caries Res 1993;27:217.
4 Emami Z, Al-Khateeb S, de Josselin de Jong E, Sundström F, Trollsås K, Angmar-Månsson B: Mineral loss in incipient caries lesions quantified with laser fluorescence and longitudinal microradiography. A methodologic study. Acta Odontol Scand 1996;54:8–13.
5 Ando M, Hall AF, Eckert GJ, Schemehorn BR, Analoui M, Stookey GK: Relative ability of laser fluorescence techniques to quantitate early mineral loss in vitro. Caries Res 1997;31:125–131.
6 Angmar-Månsson B, Al-Khateeb S, Tranaeus S: Monitoring the caries process. Optical methods for clinical diagnosis and quantification of enamel caries. Eur J Oral Sci 1996;104:480–485.
7 Bjelkhagen H, Sundström F: A clinically applicable laser luminescence method for the early detection of dental caries. IEEE J Quantum Electronics 1981;80:110–122.

8 Bjelkhagen H, Sundström F, Angmar-Månsson B, Rydén H: Early detection of enamel caries by the luminescence excited by visible light. Swed Dent J 1982;6:1–7.
9 Sundström F, Fredriksson K, Montan S, Hafström-Björkman U, Ström J: Laser-induced fluorescence from sound and carious tooth substance: Spectroscopic studies. Swed Dent J 1985;9:71–80.
10 de Josselin de Jong E, Sundström F, Westerling H, Tranaeus S, ten Bosch JJ, Angmar-Månsson B: A new method for in vivo quantification of changes in initial enamel caries with laser fluorescence. Caries Res 1995;29:2–7.
11 ten Cate JM, de Josselin de Jong E, Exterkate RAM, Sundström G, Angmar-Månsson B: Quantification of enamel demineralisation with a new portable fluorescence device, validated by microradiography (abstract 97). Caries Res 1996;30:299.
12 Al-Khateeb S, ten Cate JM, Angmar-Månsson B, de Josselin de Jong E, Sundström G, Exterkate RA, Oliveby A: Quantification of formation and remineralisation of artificial enamel lesions with a new portable fluorescence device. Adv Dent Res 1997;11:502–506.
13 Lagerweij MD, van der Veen MH, Ando M, Lukantsova L, Stookey GK: The validity and repeatability of three light-induced fluorescence systems: An in vitro study. Caries Res 1999;33:220–226.
14 ten Bosch JJ: Light scattering and related methods in caries diagnosis; in Stookey GK (ed): Early Detection of Dental Caries: Proceedings of the 1st Annual Indiana Conference. Indianapolis, Indiana University, 1996, pp 81–90.
15 de Josselin de Jong E, Hall AF, van der Veen MH: Quantitative light-induced fluorescence detection method: A Monte Carlo simulation model; in Stookey GK (ed): Early Detection of Dental Caries: Proceedings of the 1st Annual Indiana Conference. Indianapolis, Indiana University, 1996, pp 91–104.
16 Spitzer D, ten Bosch JJ: Luminescence quantum yields of sound and carious dental enamel. Calcif Tissue Res 1977;24:249–251.
17 Al-Khateeb S, Exterkate RAM, Angmar-Månsson B, ten Cate JM: Effect of acid-etching quantitatively and esthetically on remineralisation of enamel white spot lesions (abstract 21). Caries Res 1997;31:288.
18 Al-Khateeb S, Oliveby A, de Josselin de Jong E, Angmar-Månsson B: Laser fluorescence quantification of remineralisation in situ of incipient enamel lesions: Influence of fluoride supplements. Caries Res 1997;31:132–140.
19 Brinkman J, ten Bosch JJ, Borsboom PC: Optical quantification of natural caries in smooth surfaces of extracted teeth. Caries Res 1988;22:257–262.
20 Al-Khateeb S, Forsberg CM, de Josselin de Jong E, Angmar-Månsson B: A longitudinal laser fluorescence study of white spot lesions in orthodontic patients. Am J Orthod Dentofacial Orthop 1998;113:595–602.
21 Ferreira Zandoná AG, van der Veen M, Eckert GJ, Stookey GK: Clinical repeatability of light-induced fluorescence for caries detection (abstract 5). J Dent Res 1998;77:632.
22 Lagerweij MD, Beiswanger BB, van der Veen MH, Ferreira Zandoná AG, Stookey GK: Interexaminer variability of analysis of QLF images obtained from a patient (abstract 653). J Dent Res 1998; 77:713.
23 van der Veen MH, Ferreira Zandoná AG, de Josselin de Jong E, Stookey GK: Clinical evaluation of an intra-oral quantitative light-induced fluorescence camera (abstract 85). Caries Res 1998;32:296.
24 Hall AF, DeSchepper ED, van der Veen MH, de Josselin de Jong, Stookey GK: Quantitative laser fluorescence and detection of in vitro mineral changes in caries adjacent to amalgam restorations (abstract 99). Caries Res 1996;30:299.
25 Øgaard B, Rolla G, Arends J: Orthodontic appliances and enamel demineralisation. Part 1. Lesion development. Am J Orthod Dentofacial Orthop 1988;94:68–73.
26 Øgaard B, ten Bosch JJ: Regression of white spot enamel lesions: A new optical method for quantitative longitudinal evaluation in vivo. Am J Orthod Dentofacial Orthop 1994;106:238–242.
27 van der Veen MH, de Josselin de Jong E: The introduction of a new parameter ΔQ for incipient caries measurement with QLF (abstract 109), Caries Res 1999;33:318.
28 Tranaeus S, Al-Khateeb S, Björkman S, Twetman S, Angmar-Månsson B: A six-month clinical study with QLF for comparison of F varnish and professional tooth cleaning in caries-active children (abstract 71). Caries Res 1998;32:291.

29 Ferreira Zandoná AG, Isaacs RL, van der Veen M, Eckert GJ, Stookey GK: Comparison between light-induced fluorescence and clinical examinations for caries detection (abstract 86). Caries Res 1998;32:296.

30 Ando M, van der Veen MH, Schemehorn BR, Stookey GK: A comparison of quantitative light-induced fluorescence (QLF) on white-spots in permanent and deciduous enamel (abstract 130). Caries Res 1997;31:324.

31 van der Veen MH, de Josselin de Jong E, Stookey GK: Computer simulation of quantitative light-induced fluorescence (QLF) on enamel with different scattering coefficients (abstract 129). Caries Res 1997;31:323.

32 Sundström F, Hafström-Björkman U, Ström J, Angmar-Månsson B, Frostell G, Takazoe I: Evaluation of a model for short-term clinical testing of cariogenicity. J Biol Buccale 1989;17:115–120.

33 Hall AF, DeSchepper E, Ando M, Stookey GK: In vitro studies of laser fluorescence for detection and quantification of mineral loss from dental caries. Adv Dent Res 1997;11:507–514.

34 Ando M, Hall AF, Isaacs RL, Beiswanger BB, Blackman DF, Stookey GK: Comparison of clinical, quantitative laser fluorescence and dye enhanced laser fluorescence techniques for occlusal caries detection (abstract 21). Caries Res 1996;30:274.

35 Ferreira Zandoná AG, Analoui M, Schemehorn BR, Eckert GJ, Stookey GK: Laser fluorescence detection of demineralisation in artificial occlusal fissures. Caries Res 1998;32:31–40.

36 Ferreira Zandoná AG, Analoui M, Beiswanger BB, Isaacs RL, Kafrawy AH, Eckert GJ, Stookey GK: An in vitro comparison between laser fluorescence and visual examination for detection of demineralisation in occlusal pits and fissures. Caries Res 1998;32:210–218.

37 Tranaeus S, Lussi A, de Josselin de Jong E, Angmar-Månsson B: Quantification of occlusal caries: An in vitro study with laser fluorescence, electrical resistance measurement and histologic examination (abstract 101). J Dent Res 1997;76:1107.

38 Eggertsson H, Analoui M, van der Veen MH, Conzález-Cabezas C, Eckert GJ, Stookey GK: Detection of early interproximal caries in vitro using laser fluorescence, dye-enhanced laser fluorescence and direct visual examination. Caries Res 1999;33:227–233.

39 DeSchepper EJ, Hall AF, de Josselin de Jong E, Benedict S, Analoui M, Ando M, Beiswanger BB, Dixon SE, Willis GP, Stookey GK: Demineralisation detection adjacent to amalgam using quantitative laser fluorescence and dye-enhanced laser fluorescence; in Stookey GK (ed): Early Detection of Dental Caries: Proceedings of the 1st Annual Indiana Conference. Indianapolis, Indiana University, 1996, pp 165–182.

40 Tranaeus S, de Josselin de Jong E, Lussi A, Angmar-Månsson B: Quantitative light-induced fluorescence for assessment of enamel caries around fillings: A pilot study (abstract 132). Caries Res 1997; 31:324.

41 Blackman D, van der Veen M, Lagerweij M, Ando M, Stookey G: Laser fluorescence diagnosis of demineralised enamel adjacent to resin restorations (abstract 943). J Dent Res 1997;76:131.

42 Angmar-Månsson B, de Josselin de Jong E, Sundström F, ten Bosch JJ: Strategies for improving the assessment of dental fluorosis: Focus on optical techniques. Adv Dent Res 1994;8:75–79.

M.H. van der Veen, ACTA, Department of Cariology, Endodontology and Pedodontology, Louwesweg 1, NL–1066 EA Amsterdam (The Netherlands)
Tel. +31 20 5188437, Fax +31 20 6692881, E-Mail: m.vd.veen@acta.nl

Faller RV (ed): Assessment of Oral Health.
Monogr Oral Sci. Basel, Karger, 2000, vol 17, pp 163–173

Recent Advances in Methods for the Assessment of Dental Calculus – Research and Clinical Implications

Donald J. White

The Procter and Gamble Company, Cincinnati, Ohio, USA

Abstract

The diagnostic evaluation of supra- and subgingival calculus has remained an important research problem for over 40 years. The measurement of calculus remains an important objective in both research and office settings. As might be expected, the most important advances in diagnostic methods for calculus assessment have been derived from cross-fertilization from other technical disciplines including engineering, optics and computer science fields. With the new methods described herein, clinicians and researchers can look forward to important advances in our understanding of the impact of supragingival and subgingival calculus on oral health status and periodontal disease progression and in the development of treatment modalities for improved calculus control, benefiting patients and clinicians alike.

Introduction – Calculus Prevalence and Significance

Supragingival dental calculus can be found in all populations, with deposit formation strongly influenced by the frequency of routine individual and professional oral hygiene [1]. In both Western and non-Western populations, supragingival calculus represents a significant cosmetic problem. Deposits exhibit a chalky appearance with a yellow caste, making them easily visible on the teeth. Often these porous deposits acquire additional stains from diet and tobacco. In the US, the removal of supragingival calculus for cosmetic purposes during routine prophylaxis and in periodontal therapeutic procedures represents a significant health-care cost in terms of dollars and professional time and effort. In addition, tartar control toothpastes (in some form) represent over one third of US dentifrice sales and are a growing segment of global dentifrice sales.

The effects of supragingival calculus deposits on oral health varies in different populations [1]. In populations with access to routine professional dental care, supragingival calculus formation is incidental, being restricted to a limited portion of the dentition (lingual surfaces of mandibular incisors and buccal surfaces of molars – adjacent to salivary ducts) and causing no apparent health consequences [1, 2]. In populations where access to professional dental care is limited, supragingival calculus deposits are found on more teeth and in greater quantity [1, 2]. The long-term exposure of gingival tissues to extensive calculus deposits has been shown to produce localized gingival recession [3].

Subgingival calculus is prevalent in both Western and non-Western societies, although again, the quantity of subgingival calculus is found to be influenced by population access to routine professional dental care [2]. Subgingival calculus formation can be viewed as a byproduct of gingival pocket inflammation associated with early and particularly more advanced periodontal diseases [1, 4, 5]. Although scaling and root planing represent the cornerstone of phase-I periodontal therapy, the precise role of subgingival calculus deposits, e.g. cause or effect, on disease progression remains unresolved [1, 2, 6].

Determination of the precise etiologic contributions of calculus to gingival and periodontal diseases is complicated by coincident plaque formation on calculus surfaces. Available research would suggest that calculus deposits, even if they are not directly causal, certainly may contribute to the chronicity of the disease process owing to their ability to protect plaque deposits from debridement, or through direct absorption of toxic substances, such as endotoxin and lipopolysaccharides. Despite the confusion surrounding their etiologic significance in periodontal diseases, calculus deposits remain at a minimum a cosmetic nuisance and at worst a harbor for pathogenic plaque accumulation. The association between absorbed plaque and calculus requires the removal of both during professional cleaning, and the control of calculus deposition through inhibition of plaque mineralization associated with calculus hardening and adhesion remains a worthwhile therapeutic goal.

Measurement of Supra- and Subgingival Calculus – Historical Perspective

The development and application of indices for the evaluation of supra- and subgingival calculus deposits seems, at first glance, to be a simple enough task. One must simply observe or feel the deposits during probing and record observations on some sort of numeric scale, either subjective or 'semi-objective'. Despite this apparent simplicity, the development of valid and clinically relevant methods for the measurement of calculus has proven complex and difficult. This is particularly true when viewed in the larger context of applying these indices to the study of important questions such as the etiological factors important to periodontal disease, and appropriate targets for therapeutic intervention. The quantitative measurement of supra- and subgingival calculus deposits continues to play an important role in dental research.

Supragingival Calculus

Supragingival calculus has been evaluated by numerous techniques, and all have involved direct observation to some degree. The earliest common index for recording was introduced by Greene and Vermillion [7] as the Oral Hygiene Index (OHI). This index, and later variations [8], used subjective observations to separately estimate plaque, supragingival calculus and subgingival calculus on the teeth. The Periodontal Disease Index, developed by Ramfjord [9] in 1959, similarly included indices for soft and hard tooth deposits framed after the OHI, but focusing on a more limited portion of the dentition to logistically facilitate routine use in epidemiological surveys. Prior to 1969, evaluation methods for supragingival calculus were limited by relatively poor sensitivity for the assessment of calculus severity. This no doubt influenced the timely development of treatment agents aimed at reducing supragingival calculus build up. In 1969 in a series of papers, Volpe et al. [10–12] documented a more quantitative approach to the evaluation of supragingival calculus including good estimates of calculus incidence and severity. Using this method, the apical extension of supragingival calculus on the teeth is measured linearly from the base of the calculus along the gumline toward the crown of the tooth in three orientations. Measurements are made directly with a periodontal probe, marked in 1-mm increments, placed along the measured direction. The three linear measures per tooth surface can be either summed or averaged across measured surfaces to provide a composite subject calculus score. Teeth recorded with or without supragingival calculus serve as an incidence score. The Volpe-Manhold Index (VMI) has served as the clinical benchmark for supragingival calculus measurement for over three decades. The development and commercialization of modern tartar-control toothpastes was facilitated by clinical studies employing the Volpe-Manhold methodology. VMI measures have proven to correlate with calculus formed on the teeth assessed by both imaging methods and by weighing the mineralized deposits. Because the VMI is exclusively devoted to the assessment of supragingival calculus, the method would seem well suited to detailed examination of the oral health manifestations of these deposits. Unfortunately, only limited studies have taken advantage of the index in this manner. In a novel clinical design, Gaare et al. [13] used the VMI coupled with standard methods for gingivitis assessment to demonstrate that supragingival calculus deposits had little effect on gingivitis and gingival bleeding in an Indonesian population. We have observed a lack of correlation between supragingival calculus reduction provided by 'tartar-control dentifrice' and improvement in gingivitis status in repeated clinical studies [1]. More recently, a gingival recession index was developed based upon VMI design [14]. The recession index was compared with traditional VMI calculus scoring to demonstrate a correlation between localized gingival recession and supragingival calculus formation in populations lacking professional access [14, 15].

Overall, the application of the VMI measurement technique for supragingival calculus is still primarily a 'research' clinical methodology to help assess the efficacy of antitartar dentifrices and mouth rinses. Supragingival calculus is typically not recorded in regular office visits in assessments of periodontal status.

Subgingival Calculus

Subgingival calculus has historically been evaluated using combined visual-tactile techniques, and these represent components of OHI and Ramfjord indices. As a rule, subgingival measures are 'site' prevalence or incidence measures since the location of deposits has made quantitative enumeration of severity on an area or volume basis difficult if not impossible. In these measures a periodontal probe is used to gently assess tissues, measuring periodontal pocketing through subgingival penetration and measuring subgingival calculus through tactile sensation of surface roughness. In the widely used Community Periodontal Index of Treatment Needs, the calculus scoring system includes both supra- and subgingival calculus assessments, although these are not distinguished in recording [16]. The presence of calculus (supra- or subgingival) constitutes a score of 2 as opposed to bleeding alone, 1. (This scoring assumes greater pathology for the presence of calculus, with or without bleeding, than for bleeding alone. This assumption is questionable for subgingival calculus and likely to be incorrect for supragingival calculus only.) Higher scores of 3 and 4 require the gingival pocketing to be below or above 5 mm in depth.

The clinical assessment of subgingival calculus has been extensively used in efforts to track the prevalence of periodontal disease in populations. In addition, the tactile sensitivity to subgingival calculus deposits during scaling and root planing serves as a marker for the efficacy in treating these periodontal surfaces, with the objective of therapy being the development of smooth and clean surfaces by dental professionals [17]. Conventional subgingival calculus measures have only been sparingly used for the clinical assessment of possible preventive agents [18], likely due to both the limitations of grading techniques and the lack of effective therapies directed at the prevention of subgingival calculus. Care must be taken not to confuse subgingival scoring with supragingival scoring in combined studies. We have observed different results for subgingival calculus evaluated before and after supragingival (only) calculus removal (McClanahan and White, unpublished results).

Recent Advances in the Measurements of Supra- and Subgingival Calculus Deposits

Supragingival Calculus

Because the measurement of supragingival calculus is primarily applied in clinical research studies, efforts toward further optimization have been directed toward improving the sensitivity, reproducibility and, more recently, the clinical relevance of these measures.

Research to improve the sensitivity and reproducibility of visual supragingival calculus assessments have included application of image analysis techniques. Barnett et al. [19] were the first to apply imaging techniques to supragingival calculus assessments. Photographs of lingual mandibular supragingival calculus deposits taken under standardized lighting conditions were digitized and the area of calculus was calculated by computer. The area of total calculus for a panel of supragingival calculus formers was compared to conventional VMI scores and an excellent correlation ($r^2 = 0.93$, $p < 0.05$) was obtained. More recently, Dijkman et al. [20] applied computer-assisted image analysis techniques to supragingival calculus evaluations in a clinical study. VMI scores of calculus on tooth surfaces were compared to surface areas determined by computer-assisted digital image processing of photographs. Images were calibrated using known (premeasured) tooth dimensions and applying these to image standardization, thus allowing calibration to the depth of field within the image. In a crossover clinical study, the efficacy of 5% pyrophosphate dentifrice for the prevention of supragingival calculus was found to be similar for evaluations carried out by imaging techniques and conventional VMI scoring (table 1). Both theory and experience suggest that image analysis techniques can be as sensitive as VMI assessments for supragingival calculus measures. Improved measurement sensitivity is likely not the most important advantage of image processing to supragingival calculus evaluations, however. Instead, the advantages of image processing to standard VMI grader assessments are likely to be: (1) that standardized imaging measures provide a nonsubjective measure of calculus in studies, negating differences

Table 1. Comparison of VMI and computer-assisted image analysis (IA) for calculus assessments in a clinical trial[1]

Treatment	VMI calculus mm	% Reduction from placebo	IA calculus mm^2 IA field	% Reduction from placebo
Placebo	14.9	–	599	–
5% Pyrophosphate tartar-control dentifrice	10.9*	26.5	423*	29.4

* Treatment different from placebo at $p<0.05$.
[1] Three-month double-blind crossover design.

in studies owing to variable examiner sensitivities and application of VMI, and (2) that standardized imaging measures provide a permanent quantitative record of assessments in clinical studies. Although the ease of training of VMI examiners and experience with these techniques still encourage more traditional examinations, it is nevertheless likely that the straightforward application of modern image-processing software will encourage the increased use of image analysis for supragingival calculus assessments.

A completely new approach to the evaluation of supragingival calculus was published by our laboratories in a series of articles in 1996. The rationale behind the research was that supragingival calculus formation in Western populations presented a nuisance in two aspects: the cosmetic appearance on the teeth, and the efforts required in debridement. Indeed, we reasoned that the inconvenience associated with supragingival calculus removal was likely a more important aspect of calculus formation than appearance on the teeth, since patients receiving regular dental cleanings most typically form calculus in locations not easily visible (lingual surfaces of mandibular incisors and buccal surfaces of maxillary molars) [21]. Our laboratories developed a transducer-modified dental scaler, called the Quanticalc, which measures forces generated at the tooth surfaces in scaling calculus debris from the teeth [22]. The transducer-modified scaler and the computer-controlled clinical device are shown in figure 1. Clinical studies established that the Quanticalc provides valid measures of the combined quantity and clinical manifestations (removal effort) associated with calculus formation and the professional debridement required. The Quanticalc has been used in controlled, double-blind, clinical studies to compare the efficacy of tartar-control toothpastes containing various ingredients. In one large-scale trial, the clinical efficacy of a dentifrice containing 5% pyrophosphate was compared with that of a placebo (nontartar control)

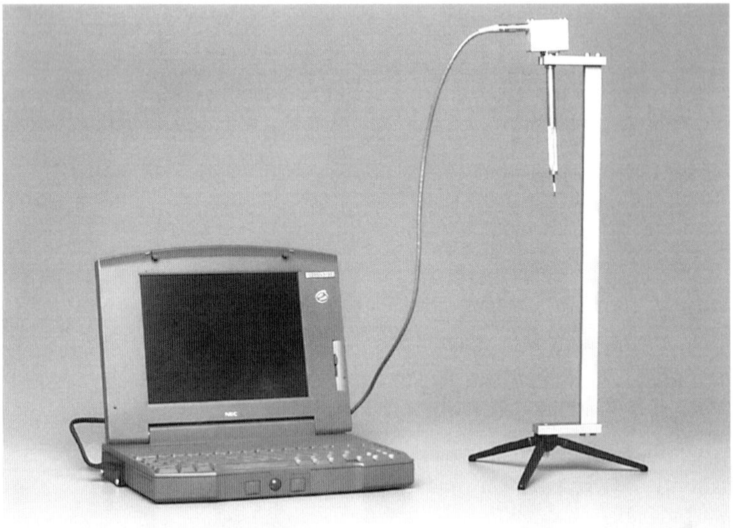

Fig. 1. QC scaler clinical unit as used today. Computer control of transducer-modified scaler permits real-time collection of scaling information on a tooth-site basis. Scaler handpiece with curette is shown on the right.

dentifrice and a dentifrice containing a combination of 1.3% pyrophosphate and 1.5% Gantrez copolymer [23]. Results, summarized in table 2, show that the two tartar-control toothpastes provide comparable efficacy for prevention of tartar buildup between dental cleanings, as measured by the traditional VMI surface area index. However, the calculus which formed between dental cleanings behaved quite differently in response to efforts toward removal. As shown in table 2, the efficacy of the two tartar-control dentifrices in facilitating easier calculus debridement differed by a factor of 2. This suggests that some tartar-control agents might exhibit improved efficacy by making calculus much easier to clean for professionals, making dental cleanings simpler and more comfortable for patients.

It is expected that measures of supragingival tartar-control activity in future studies may include scaling efficiency evaluations using Quanticalc devices as a standard for efficacy. Moreover, the Quanticalc device itself may prove useful in hygienist and dentist training. The evaluation of treatment agents for efficacy in terms of prophylaxis effort may be preferred to simple measures of tooth surface area covered by calculus. Scaling procedures in regular office visits create mild discomfort for most patients and the provision of easier dental cleanings is strongly motivating. Further, the reductions in professional efforts associated with manual debridement of supragingival cal-

Table 2. Comparison of VMI index and Quanticalc index evaluations of tartar-control dentifrice efficacy: 6-month clinical results[1]

Treatment	VMI calculus mm	% Reduction from placebo	QC prophylaxis force to clean kg	% Reduction from placebo
Placebo	17.83[a]		11.79[a]	
Tartar-control dentifrice containing 1.3% pyrophosphate and 1.5% CoPolymer	14.74[b]	17.3	10.03[b]	15.0
Tartar-control dentifrice containing 5% pyrophosphate	14.71[b]	17.8	8.55[c]	27.5

Treatment group designations refer to statistical comparisons at $p < 0.05$, ANCOVA, $a \neq b \neq c$.
[1] n = 215–219 per group; parallel design double-blind study.

culus may pay dividends in cost, time and professional fatigue [21]. Additional studies with the Quanticalc scaler toward these ends have evaluated the efficacy of scaling gels and compared the efficiency of professional technique in calculus debridement [24, 25].

Subgingival Calculus

The quantitative measurement of subgingival calculus is a daunting proposition. These highly mineralized deposits can be found below the gingival margin throughout the dentition. Deposits form on all surfaces (buccal, proximal) including areas below furcations in severely compromised teeth. Although proximal subgingival calculus deposits are often discernible in radiographs, these methods have proven unreliable as research tools and provide only supplementary information to standard clinical examinations [26]. Similarly, tactile probing has proven of only modest specificity and sensitivity in clinical examinations [27]. The sustained difficulty in the development of quantitative measures for subgingival calculus deposits has strongly impacted our ability to establish the etiological significance of these deposits, develop new treatment modalities for subgingival calculus prevention and improve the overall effectiveness of phase-I periodontal therapy (scaling and root planing). Fortunately, research continues against this complex objective.

With respect to direct imaging, that is viewing of subgingival deposits, the most promising new research would appear to be the application of fiberoptic systems. Fiberoptic illumination and transillumination has proven effective in identifying subgingival calculus in proximal sites and the use of this technique in combination with papilla reflection have resulted in improved scaling efficiencies [28, 29]. More recently, the DentalView Incorporated has developed a PerioView® system which combines fiberoptic technology found in numerous medical applications (angioscopes, neuroscopes, etc.) with commonly used dental instruments [30]. The manufacturer of the PerioView® system indicates that the system provides the diagnostic ability to evaluate the presence and type of dental calculus without surgical flapping. Specially designed hand instruments allow fiberoptics to be used during the actual scaling procedure. Disposable protective sheaths permit simple, cost-effective and sterile observations in multiple sites and patients, and the probing unit can be combined with an infusion pump to wash areas clear of debris to facilitate easier viewing. A direct video/hard copy of examination results can be obtained for permanent records. To this author's knowledge, the PerioView® system, if proven to work practically, will be the first reproducible diagnostic technique to permit research clinicians and periodontal practitioners to directly view patients' teeth subgingivally. From a research standpoint, the technique may provide the diagnostic ability to evaluate the presence/absence of subgingival calculus without subjective and imprecise tactile measures and without surgical flapping. These examinations may in principal include teeth with furcations. Commercially available in December 1998, the PerioView® system may represent a major advance in the diagnostic measurement of subgingival calculus. It will be interesting to monitor the progress of researchers and periodontal practitioners in the application of this device to their work.[1]

In addition to improved visual evaluation techniques research advances have also been recently made in the tactile assessment of subgingival calculus. Jeffcoat et al. [31] have developed an acoustic sensor-modified periodontal probe which is effective in surface roughness associated with subgingival calculus. Preliminary measurements in vitro and in vivo suggest reasonable sensitivity and specificity for the detection of proximal subgingival calculus. Zappa et al. [32] have developed a transducer-modified scaler which measures forces applied by the therapist in scaling and root planing. The device can be used to monitor the effort required to complete scaling and root planing as well as the efficiency of subgingival therapy. Likewise, we (unpublished results) have applied the Quanticalc device to subgingival calculus removal and successfully recorded forces developed in scaling and root planing debridement. While perhaps not as 'efficient' as direct viewing, the application of these 'transducer'-modified scalers may assist in improving the efficiency of scaling and root planing procedures, as well as serving as potential diagnostic tools.

[1] DentalView Inc. and PerioView® are not affiliated with the Procter and Gamble Co.. Researchers interested in the device can visit the company's website at DentalView.com.

As stated earlier, measures of subgingival calculus are complicated by the fact that calculus can form on all surfaces below the gingival margin. Even with the advances described herein, the three dimensional tracking of deposits during a whole mouth examination remains a substantial undertaking. On the other hand, it is likely that advanced methods of subgingival calculus detection can finally permit at least the routine assessment of calculus presence/absence throughout the dentition. This alone may be sufficient for use in both practice-based and clinical research settings. The application of advanced fiberoptic direct-viewing technology and transducer-modified scaler/probe technologies offers hope that future clinical and epidemiological research may provide deeper insights into the role of subgingival calculus in periodontal disease advancement and facilitate the development of treatments for its prevention and removal.

References

1 White DJ: Dental calculus: Recent insights into occurrence, formation, prevention, removal and oral health effects of supragingival and subgingival deposits. Eur J Oral Sci 1997;105:508–522.
2 Anerud A, Loe H, Boysen H: The natural history and clinical course of calculus formation in man. J Clin Periodontol 1991;18:160–170.
3 van Palenstein-Helderman WH, Lembariti BS, van der Veijden GA, van't Hof MA: Gingival recession and its association with calculus in subjects deprived of prophylactic dental care. J Clin Peridontol 1998;25:106–111.
4 Mandel ID, Gaffar A: Calculus revisited. A review. J Clin Periodontol 1986;13:249–257.
5 Mandel ID: Calculus update: Prevalence, pathogenicity and prevention. J Am Dent Assoc 1995; 126:573–580.
6 Zappa U: Factors determining the outcome of scaling and root planing. Probe 1992;26:152–159.
7 Greene JC, Vermillion JR: The oral hygiene index: A method for classifying oral hygiene status. J Am Dent Assoc 1960;61:171–177.
8 Greene JC, Vermillion JR: The simplified oral hygiene index. J Am Dent Assoc 1964;68:7–11.
9 Ramfjord SP: Indices for prevalence and incidence of periodontal disease. J Periodontol 1959;30:51–64.
10 Volpe AR, Manhold JH, Hazen SP: In vivo calculus assessment. Part I: A method and its examiner reproducibility. J Periodontol 1965;36:292–298.
11 Volpe AR, Manhold JH, Hazen SP: In vivo calculus assessment. Part II: A comparison of scoring techniques. J Periodontol 1965;36:299–304.
12 Volpe AR, Manhold JH, Hazen SP: In vivo calculus assessment. Part III: Scoring techniques, rate of calculus formation, partial mouth exams vs Fullmouth exams and intra-examiner reproducibility. Periodontics 1967;5:184–193.
13 Gaare D, Rolla G, Aryadi FJ, Van der Ouderaa F: Improvement of gingival health by toothbrushing in individuals with large amounts of calculus. J Clin Periodontol 1990;17:38–41.
14 Volpe AR, Triratana T, Rustogi KN: Development of a system to assess visible and hidden gingival recession. J Clin Dent 1991;3(suppl B):B6–B11.
15 Rustogi KN, Triratana T, Lindhe J, Volpe AR: The association between supragingival calculus deposits and the extent of gingival recession in a sample of Thai children and teenagers. J Clin Dent 1991;3(suppl B):B1–B5.
16 Ainamo J, Barmes D, Beagrie G, Cutress T, Martin J, Sardo-Infirri J: Development of the World Health Organization (WHO) Community Periodontal Index of Treatment Needs (CPITN). Int Dent J 1982;32:281–291.

17 Drisko CL, Killoy WJ: Scaling and root planing: Removal of calculus and subgingival organisms. Current Opin Dent 1991;1:74–80.
18 Suomi JD, Horowitz HS, Barbano JP, Spolski VW, Heifetz SB: A clinical trial of a calculus inhibitory dentifrice. J Periodontol 1974;45:139–145.
19 Barnett ML, Charles CH, Gilman RM, Bartels LL: Correlation between Volpe-Manhold calculus index scores and actual calculus area. Clin Prev Dent 1989;11:3–5.
20 Dijkman AG, Sokroos I, McCormack L, Arends J, Cox ER, Bacca L, Sturzenberger OP, White DJ: The application of image analysis in Standardized Calculus Assessments (abstract 469). J Dent Res 1994;73:160.
21 White DJ: Tartar control: Assessment of patient benefit and professional scaling advantages. J Clin Dent 1996;7:27–31.
22 White DJ, Cox ER, Arends J, Hieborg JH, Leydsman H, Wieringa DW, Dijkman AG, Ruben JR: Instruments and methods for the quantitative measurement of factors affecting hygienist/dentist efforts during scaling and root planing of the teeth. J Clin Dent 1996;7:32–40.
23 White DJ, McClanahan SF, Lanzalaco AC, Cox ER, Bacca L, Perlich MA, Campbell SL, Schiff T, Stains A: The comparative efficacy of two commercial tartar control dentifrices in preventing calculus development and facilitating easier dental cleanings. J Clin Dent 1996;7:58–64.
24 Arends J, Dijkman AG, White DJ, Cox ER: Effects of a scaling gel on forces developed in debridement of supragingival calculus determined by means of a transducer modified dental scaler: The Quanticalc. J Clin Dent 1996;7:50–53.
25 White DJ, Cox ER, Bacca L, Lanzalaco AC, Montgomery RM, Coyle-Rees M, Beiswanger BB, Mau M, Arends J: A quanticalc clinical comparison of professional efficiency in manual supragingival calculus debridement. J Clin Dent 1996;7:54–57.
26 Buchanan SA, Jenderseck RS, Granet MA, Kircos LT, Chambers DW, Robertson PB: Radiographic detection of dental calculus. Clinical comparison of professional efficiency in manual supragingival calculus debridement. J Clin Dent 1996;7:54–57.
27 Bader HI: Scaling and root planing: Its role in contemporary periodontal therapy. Compendium 1993;14:436–449.
28 Johnson GK, Reinhardt RA, Tussing GJ, Krejci RF: Fiber optic probe augmented sonic scaling versus conventional sonic scaling. J Periodontology 1989;60:131–136.
29 Reinhardt RA, Johnson GK, Tussing GJ: Root paning with interdental papilla reflection and fiber optic illumination. J Periodontol 1985;56:721–726.
30 DentalView – PerioView System Product Promotional Material. Irvine, DentalView, Dec 29, 1998.
31 Jeffcoat RL, Chaves E, Reddy MS, Jeffcoat MK: Electronic calculus detector – Clinical use and validation (abstract 2309). J Dent Res 1994;73:390.
32 Zappa U, Cadosch J, Simona C, Graf H, Case D: In vivo scaling and root planing forces. J Periodontol 1991;62:335–340.

Dr. Donald J. White, Procter and Gamble HCRC,
PO Box 8006, Mason, Ohio 45040-8006 (USA)
Tel. +1 513 622 2205, Fax +1 513 622 0413, E-Mail white.dj.1@pg.com

Faller RV (ed): Assessment of Oral Health.
Monogr Oral Sci. Basel, Karger, 2000, vol 17, pp 174–189

Characterization and Validation of Diagnostic Methods

Jaap J. ten Bosch[a], *Birgit Angmar-Månsson*[b]

[a] Department of Biomedical Engineering, University of Groningen, the Netherlands, and

[b] Department of Cariology and Endodontology, Karolinska Institute, Huddinge, Sweden

Abstract

Diagnosis is defined as the determination of disease, but not as the determination of the signs and symptoms thereof. The use of modern diagnostic methodology in the clinic is hampered by cost considerations and by the still widespread belief that, e.g. caries lesions and periodontal breakdown are irreversible processes that need to be detected and treated invasively as early as possible, their measurement thus being irrelevant. Modern instrumental and quantitative methods allow early detection and introduction of noninvasive preventive measures to control the development of the disease. Such methods are also very beneficial in clinical research as they may describe the speed of progress or regress of disease. In epidemiology, such methods reduce the classical problem of calibration of observers. Repeatability, reproducibility, accuracy and validity are defined as method-characterizing quantities, for which examples are given. To express the validity of quantitative methods compared with a quantitative gold standard, the use of scatter plots and correlation and regression methods is suggested. Validation of a dichotomous method with a dichotomous gold standard in terms of sensitivity and specificity is discussed. To validate a quantitative method with a dichotomous gold standard, the receiver operating characteristic curve is suggested, with the requirement that the cutoff value should be determined in relation to the use of the method. However, preferably a quantitative method should not be reduced to a dichotomous one by using a cutoff value, but instead all available information should be used by the diagnostician. It is argued that the use of a secondary standard instead of the accepted gold standard usually leads to inadequate results, even when the validity of the secondary standard is known. Finally, it is argued that the choice of a gold standard is a matter of reasoning and weighing of arguments and not of following a prescribed procedure.

Introduction

Diagnosis is defined in dictionaries as the determination of diseases by their signs and symptoms. Thus, it is not the determination of the signs and symptoms themselves. In practical clinical work in, e.g. caries and periodontal disease this definition of diagnosis translates to the evaluation of the disease activity. This evaluation requires clinical examination and quantification of all factors associated with the pathogenesis of caries and periodontal disease, respectively. It is inadequate to restrict the diagnostic examinations to the momentary determinations of lesions, cavities, periodontal pockets, bone loss, and similar signs of disease. The use of the disease-oriented definition of diagnosis will not only require more diagnostic work, it will often also require a change in thinking by the diagnosing clinician. Aside from practical clinical work, diagnosis is also applied in clinical research and epidemiology or screening. In those cases it may have more restricted meanings.

Diagnostic Methods

Traditionally, diagnosis is restricted to the momentary situation and is done only by 'clinical judgement' by an experienced dentist or physician. This still is the start of the investigation of the cause of a health complaint. A patient coming with a wish or complaint to a doctor or dentist is consciously or subconsciously judged with the 'clinical view'. This view is then usually complemented with an anamnesis and a physical or oral examination. On the basis of the findings or the absence thereof, it may be decided to determine other parameters such as salivary flow, blood constituents and/or the making of nonvisual images by X-ray, ultrasound, nuclear techniques, etc. Often, the results of an implementation of a 'best guess' therapy provide additional information.

In general dentistry, common methods to determine the momentary situation are the clinical examination, the use of light, probes and pocket probes, palpation, percussion, methods of vitality testing, and the making of some type of X-ray image. In orthodontics the measuring of size parameters of the skull, face and jaws is indispensable. In oral surgery, advanced imaging methods like magnetic resonance imaging and positron emission tomography, and methods of pathology are used.

The reasons for the limited use of additional methods in general dentistry are at least twofold. First of all, there is the matter of cost. Dental problems are not life threatening, and thus cost is a major factor in dental care. Diagnostic methods in restorative dentistry and periodontology will only be used when they pay themselves in terms of a decrease in treatment costs or in time benefit to the dentist and patient. Secondly, there is the matter of thinking. Dental caries, and to a lesser extent also periodontal disease, were until recently considered diseases with an irreversible process. This implied that a prediction of the progress was futile: the progress had to be stopped by a restorative measure as soon as possible. Even in cases of doubt the restoration of a possibly sound surface was considered to be preferable over neglecting the restoration of an early lesion. Accordingly, generations of dentists were trained that a good determination of the present status of the condition was adequate. To do so, a visual and tactile examination, supplemented by X-ray images and a pocket probe, sufficed.

Presently, in dental caries the restriction to the momentary situation is no longer considered adequate. The progress of carious lesions is slower and cavitation occurs much later than one or two decades ago. This is mainly an effect of fluoride-containing dentifrice. At least incipient caries lesions can be arrested and possibly remineralized by proper fluoride treatment and oral hygiene. This shifts the decision-making balance towards a much more conservative attitude, thus the diagnosis becomes more important in cases of doubt. The diagnostic question has changed from a description of the present state towards the prediction of the future progress. This makes it relevant to predict progress on the basis of quantitative determination and monitoring of the disease. Such monitoring will also enable feedback to the patient regarding preventive measures such as a change in dietary habits or oral hygiene.

Additional need for quantitative and objective methods comes from clinical research and epidemiology. In clinical research, quantitative methods may describe the speed of progress or regress of disease and will thus enable the effect of influencing measures in a quantitative way. This hopefully leads to a less confounded analysis on a shorter term than, caries research taken as an example, the classical counting of the number of teeth, lesions and fillings made by a treating dentist. In epidemiology, the classical exercise of calibration of observers may be simplified by methods that 'objectively' measure and record the status of disease.

As a result, much laboratory and, to a lesser extent, clinical work has been done to develop new diagnostic methods and to improve or simplify older ones [1–4].

A diagnostic tool that measures a single symptom is never flawless, although often more reliable than a clinical judgement of that symptom. To a major or minor extent, any measurement is subject to influences by the user/observer, to changes in the environment (temperature, humidity, light level, instabilities in the power source, etc.), to internal changes in the instrument itself (ageing of light sources, optical fibers, electrical components, etc.). Further, all biological quantities are subject to variations, which usually have a normal distribution. Thus, outliers occur that correspond to a healthy situation. This implies that any observation should be combined with other observations, at least the 'clinical judgement'. Never should any instrument or measurement be considered as the only decisive argument when its results contrast with other findings and/or common sense. Then the discrepancy should be investigated and a conclusion drawn from the entire pool of information. Further, such flaws and the susceptibility to unknown factors require that any method is properly characterized in specifications and is validated, i.e. the diagnostic value is determined.

The view on diagnosis outlined above has the consequence that diagnostic methods should preferably be quantitative rather than qualitative. In other words: preferable methods produce a number rather than a dichotomy: a yes/no outcome. There are two arguments: first a dichotomy provides only crude information that is inadequate for time-dependent monitoring of the course of disease. Secondly, a dichotomous method tends to be decisive or at least overvalued, certainly when it is the only instrumental and therefore 'objective' method in an entire diagnostic process. This undesirably will reduce the necessary thinking about discrepancies and conclusions. Most undesirable is to discard information by reducing a quantitative method to a qualitative one by defining a cutoff value. This deprives the diagnostician from valuable information. Nevertheless, qualitative methods being available and common practice, we will pay attention to their validation in the following sections.

In these sections, we will first consider the parameters that may be used to characterize any method of measurement. Then we will consider validation of a method, using different sections for different types of methods. Finally, we will devote a section to the question how improvement of methods can be combined with validation. The reasoning will be illustrated with examples from the literature the authors are most familiar with. This is not an attempt to provide a comprehensive review.

Characterization of Methods.

Any diagnostic method has to be tested. That is, three quantities have to be determined that characterize variation of results. For methods that produce continuous variables, these quantities are standard deviations of the results of three experiments. For methods that produce results in categories, most simple: dichotomies, these quantities are values of Cohen's kappa, κ. κ may range from -1 to $+1$, with perfect agreement of the observations $\kappa = 1$, and without any relation between the observations, $\kappa = 0$. Sometimes, e.g. [5] these quantities are specified as a percentage of results lying within a specified interval. Such a percentage can be recalculated to a standard deviation value.

Repeatability is the capacity of a method to produce the same results over and over again on the same object or subject and under the same circumstances. Although a clear definition, its measurement is not so easy to realize: many methods of measurement alter the object of measurement; biological objects change from day to day and so do the environmental conditions. Investigators should analyze the situation under study and then do, as well as they can, repeated measurements.

Reproducibility is the capacity of a method to produce the same results under different circumstances. Often the way a method and/or the object or subject is handled by the observer is a cause of variation. To determine the reproducibility, conditions should be varied as much as possible and the resulting standard deviation of results determined. The value obtained is then usually larger than the repeatability, since there are more sources of variation. When in such a variation only a single observer is involved, the intra-observer reproducibility is found. When more observers are involved, the variation process leads to the inter-observer reproducibility. This, similarly, is usually larger than the intra-observer reproducibility. It is fruitful to determine the causes of the variations. Taking many measurements and recording the conditions, observers, sequential number of measurement in the 'same' condition, etc., can do this. Then these data with the results of the measurements are fed into a statistical program for analysis of variance, which then produces the contributions of the different sources of variation. In either case, consultation of a methodologist/statistician before the measurements are done, is advisable.

Of course, a description of a method 'looks better' when the variation in its results is small. Standardizing the circumstances of measurement contributes to a small variation. The pitfall here is that in doing so the generalizability is decreased. For instance, when a method is strongly dependent on conditions of illumination, these may be standardized to 'normal daylight under a clouded sky' to make the reproducibility better. However, there are many places on earth where this condition is rare and thus the method cannot be generalized to such places. As another example, handling a method by a single operator reduces the variation to the intra-observer reproducibility, but data thus obtained are useless to anyone else, as they cannot use that specific operator.

The accuracy describes how well the method determines the quantity that it is meant to determine. Thus, in diagnosis the term accuracy is restricted to measuring a quantity that is a sign or symptom of disease such as pocket depth, mineral loss, plaque coverage, leukin concentrations, etc. Accuracy usually has a systematic component, i.e. a constant difference or ratio between the true and measured value of the quantity, and a stochastic component, i.e. although the reproducibility is good there is a random difference between the true and measured value.

Validation, General

Validity refers to the diagnostic value of the method. That is: the validity of a method describes the relation of its results with the determination of the disease. Often, but undesirably, the word validation is also used for determination of the accuracy. This is a more restricted meaning: the comparison of the outcome of two methods that both measure the same quantity.

In either the full or the restricted meaning, validation of a method is the comparison of the outcome of the method with a 'gold standard' of diagnosis or of measurement, respectively. This gold standard is to be chosen by the investigator of the method. The choice should be made such that the gold standard as closely as possible relates to the aim of use of the method. For instance: when a diagnostic method for the activity of the caries process is to be used to predict progress or regress of a caries lesion, the gold standard should be progress and regress. This could be quantified as the period until cavitation or undetectability of the lesions, respectively. This is not easily applicable, e.g. because such an investigation could be considered unethical. Thus, usually more indirect methods are used as a secondary standard. In this example perhaps the loss of mineral from, or the gain of mineral by, the volume of the specified lesion. This strengthens the remark that there is no prescription on what the gold standard should be: it is matter of choice.

Validation of Methods that Produce Continuous Parameters by Comparison with a Gold Standard that Is also Continuous

In this section we consider the case in which the method to be validated and the gold standard both determine a variable that can have many values. Often these variables are continuous; at least they are ranking variables. In other fields of science the validation in this case is called 'calibration'. Both methods are applied in the same conditions to a sample of subjects or objects. The sample should have a large variation in values of the gold standard variable, but it does not have to be representative of the population from which it is drawn. The most informative way of presenting the resulting information is a scatter plot. In such a plot the 'true' value is plotted horizontally, the value obtained with the new method vertically. An example is given by Biesbrock [6] in his figure 4. Another example is shown in figure 1. Ideally, there is no variation of the points around a straight or curved line. In practice, there always is and statistics have to come in to further summarize the information. The statistics are simpler when the line is straight: a linear dependence. However, often there is no theoretical background indicating such a simple linear dependence. Such a background is often assumed, which is only permitted when the points in the scatter plot do not indicate a nonlinear dependence between the two methods. In other words: when the points do not clearly indicate a curved line. Sometimes a transformation of the results of the new method, such as logarithmization, may achieve a linear dependence.

When a linear dependence may be assumed the correlation between the two methods can be calculated using the product-moment correlation coefficient, r. Then also linear regression analysis may be applied and a 95% confidence interval of the resulting regression line calculated (fig. 1). Attention is to be given to the question whether or not the regression line should include the origin of the scatter plot (fig. 1). Often, the cloud of scatter points or a regression calculation indicates that the regression line should not include the origin although first thought or theory indicates it should. Then a careful analysis of possible confounding factors that would cause systematic deviations in the results of either method is needed. When a linear dependence may not be assumed, a rank correlation coefficient and nonlinear regression models have to be employed.

Calculation of the 95% confidence interval for the regression line is particularly useful when the new method is to be applied to individual cases, e.g. in patient care. For each result of the new method the lines then indicate what the 95% confidence interval of the value of the gold standard is. Figure 1a shows this: for a result of 15% fluorescence loss the 95% confidence interval of the true ΔZ runs from 0.027 to 0.040 kg/m^2. As in this case, this interval usually is unpleasantly high. High values of the correlation coefficient, such as $r = 0.9$ or higher, are needed for individual application of a new method. In figure 1, $r = 0.76$.

Validation of Methods that Produce Dichotomies

In this situation the gold standard and the new method are applied to a sample of subjects or objects. Only two results are possible: 'sound' or 'diseased'. The gold standard gives the 'true' value. Common parameters are the sensitivity and specificity, determined by assigning a status by the new

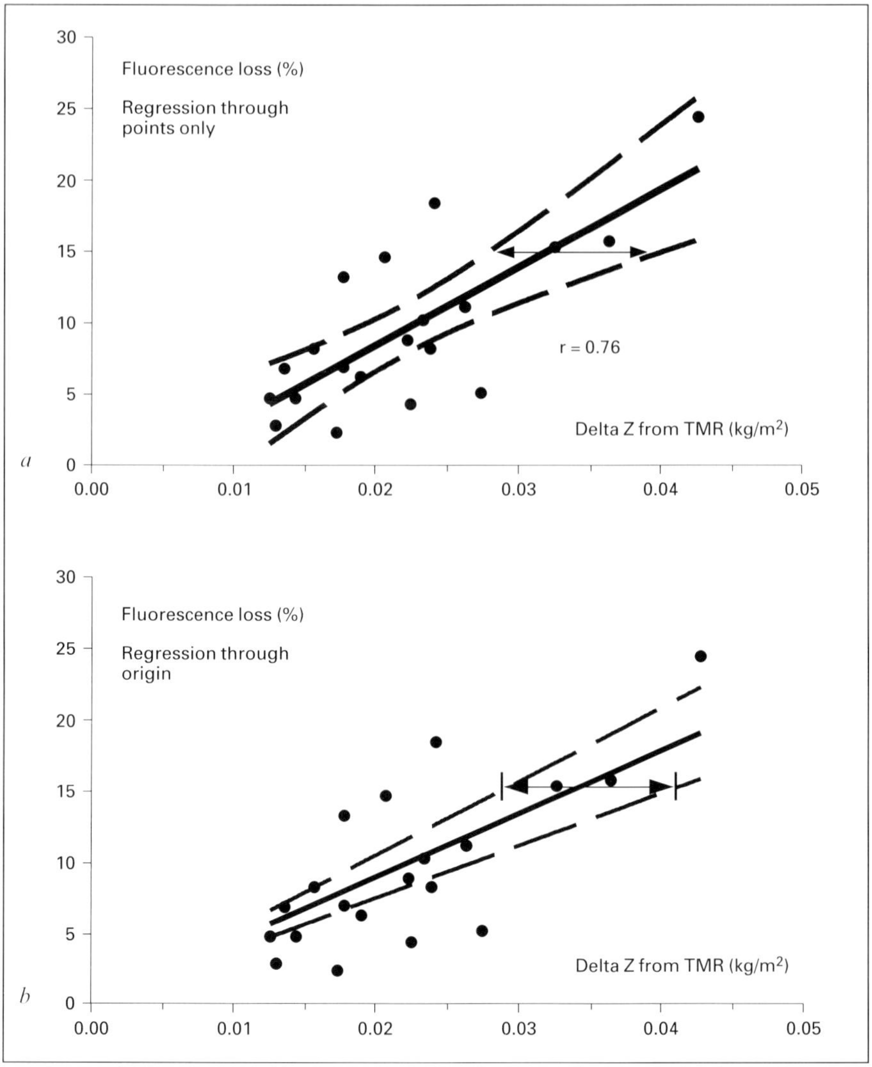

Fig. 1. Scatter plot of the validation of quantitative light-induced fluorescence (QLF) by transversal microradiography (TMR) of a section of the lesion (data from Al-Khateeb et al. [14, fig. 6]). The fluorescence loss measured by QLF is given on the vertical; the mineral loss ΔZ in kg/m^2 by TMR is given on the horizontal. *a* A line of linear regression is added. *b* A line of linear regression that goes through the origin is added. The area between the dashed lines is the area of the 95% confidence interval for the respective regression lines. The lines with arrows indicate the 95% confidence interval of true lesion depth for a lesion in which fluorescence loss = 15%.

method to the subjects in the sample. The 'true' status is determined by the gold standard method. The sensitivity and specificity are then defined as:

Sensitivity ≡ fraction of truly diseased subjects that is assigned as 'diseased' by the new method;

Specificity ≡ fraction of truly sound subjects that is assigned as 'sound' by the new method.

In doing so, it is most important that the sample is representative of the population the methods are to be applied to. Since this usually involves a lot of measurements on obviously sound or obviously diseased subjects and thus a lot of work, this rule is often violated. Nevertheless, this rule should be followed as previous work [7] showed that the results of a test are strongly dependent upon the composition of the sample. The following example makes the cause of this clear.

Suppose one selects a sample that is composed only of obviously diseased and obviously sound subjects. Then both the new method and the gold standard will give equal assignments on all subjects in the sample. Both sensitivity and specificity will be 1.0. However, no one is interested in a method that only works on obviously diseased or sound subjects. Suppose now that a sample with only marginally diseased subjects is used. Then the use of both the new method and gold standard will probably yield a sensitivity and a specificity of around 0.5, as on such a sample the factor 'guess' will play a large role. Thus, the result of a testing of a new method is strongly influenced by the composition of the sample that is used for the testing. The theoretical basis for this fact is that the assignment 'diseased' or 'sound' is essentially based upon a continuous variable such as severity of a symptom, or (in case of a true dichotomy such as gender or pregnancy) probability of correctness of assignment by the observer.

Thus, the only correct sample is the one that is truly representative of the population for which the test results should be valid. This implies random sampling, possibly through some more intricate method like block sampling. Most often this is not possible or requires too much effort. Then the report should include the method to compose the sample in comparison with the (estimated) composition of the population. When the frequency distribution of the underlying continuous variable in the sample is known, it should be given as well.

Validation of Methods that Produce Continuous Parameters by Comparison with a Gold Standard that Is a Dichotomy

Often, a new method is a quantitative one where the gold standard method is a dichotomy. Then the question arises as to how the new method is to be related to the gold standard. Such a relation can easily lead to abuse of the new method as it promotes the reduction of its use to the determination of a dichotomous result: sound or diseased. This reduction is particularly probable when the new method is an instrumental one and therefore more objective than the presumably subjective gold standard, even when used in its reduced form. We have argued in an earlier section that such a reduction of information is undesirable. We have proposed that all information about the disease status, obtained from new and old methods, should be collected by the diagnosing dentist and used as ingredients in a process of careful analysis.

However, the relation between the new method and the standard used previously is to be investigated. This is done by constructing a receiver operating characteristic (ROC) curve. To do so, a widely varying sample of subjects is subjected to the gold standard and the method to be tested. Although desirable, the sample does not have to be representative of the population. For each subject, the gold standard yields an assignment 'diseased' or 'sound'; the new method yields a number. Within the range of possible outcomes of the new method a 'cutoff value' is chosen, which reduces the obtained numbers to assignments 'diseased' or 'sound'. To avoid ambiguity, this cutoff value should always be between two numbers that can be the result of the new method. These assignments produce a sensitivity and specificity of the new method. Naturally, these will depend on the cutoff value. For a cutoff value chosen near the 'diseased' end of the range of numbers that the new method may yield, the large majority of assignments will be 'sound' and thus the specificity will be high. Adversely, for a cutoff value chosen near the 'sound' end of the range of numbers, the large majority of assignments will be 'diseased'; and the sensitivity will be high. These calculations are performed for many choices of cutoff value, which leads to many pairs of sensitivity and specificity. Finally, (sensitivity) is plotted versus (1– specificity) in a square plot, any point corresponding to another cutoff value. The line through the points is the ROC curve.

Figure 2 illustrates this process for the comparison, i.e. validation, of the electric caries monitor (ECM) [8]. This method is intended to indicate the severity of caries lesions in pits and fissures. It measures the conductivity of the tooth between a blunt electrode and the body; the result is expressed as a value between –1 and 13. Values 0 and lower correspond to sound enamel, 11 and higher to a severe (pulp or deep dentinal) caries lesion. When the chosen cutoff value is low, say –0.5, almost all teeth will lead to an ECM reading above the cutoff, and thus be assigned as 'diseased'. Thus certainly all truly diseased teeth will be assigned as diseased and thus the sensitivity is high. Since also many truly (according to the gold standard) sound teeth will be assigned 'diseased', the specificity will be low and thus (1– specificity) is high. The corresponding point is in the top right corner of figure 2. Conversely,

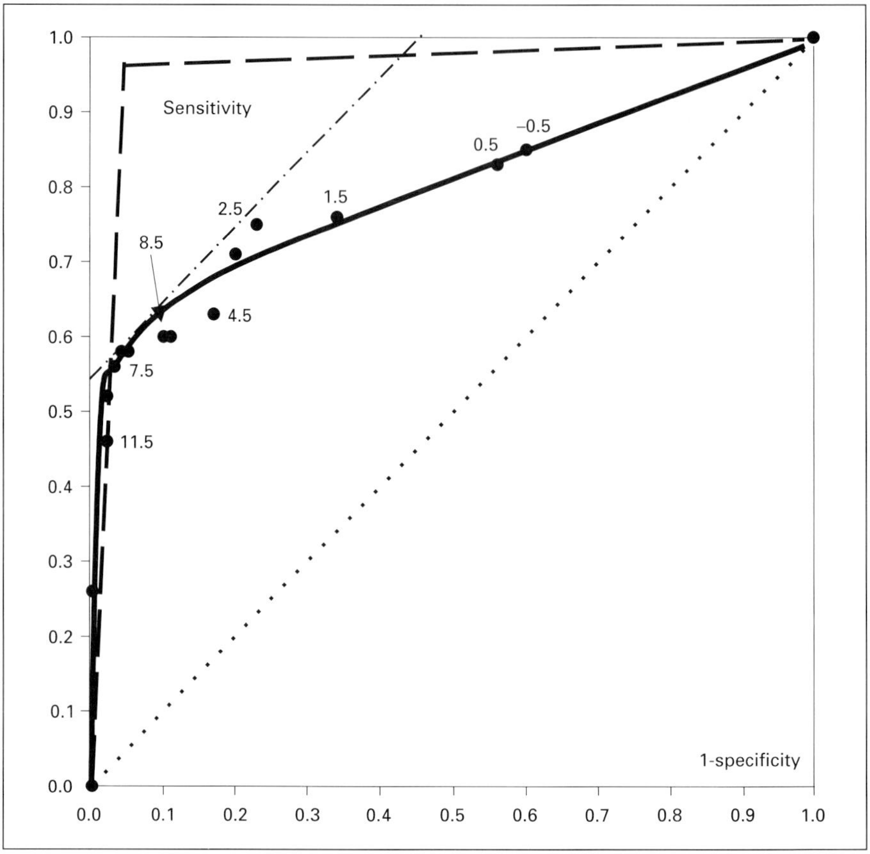

Fig. 2. ROC-curve constructed for the validation of the electric caries monitor (ECM) as done by Huysmans et al. (1998). The ECM gives integer readings in a range of –1 to 13.0. Low values correspond to sound enamel, high ones to a severe (deep dentinal with or without pulp involvement) crown caries lesion. In this study, several versions of the method were compared. Points given here refer to the so-called 'site method'. Histology is used as the gold standard. The points correspond to different cutoff values as indicated. The full line is the 'best guess' of the ROC curve. More in general, the dashed line shows the curve for a method that corresponds closely to the gold standard: both sensitivity and specificity can be nearly equal to 1. The dotted line will be found when a new method is no better than a random assignment. Accordingly, the area under the ROC curve is often used as a measure of quality; it may range from 0.5 to 1.0. In the ECM case, it amounts to 0.82. The dash-dot line is the 45° tangent to the ROC curve; the meeting point indicates the preferable cutoff (i.e. 8.0) when there is no preference for a high sensitivity or specificity at the cost of the other quantity.

when the cutoff value is 12.5, almost all teeth will have an ECM reading below 12.5 and be assigned as 'sound'. Thus certainly all truly sound teeth will be assigned as sound and thus the specificity is high. Since also many teeth with caries lesions will be assigned 'sound', the sensitivity will be low. The point is in the lower left corner of figure 2. For inbetween cutoff values, points are on a curved line. An ROC curve that approaches the upper left corner (dashed line, fig. 2) will produce a result that is identical to the result of the gold standard, provided the cutoff is chosen at that point in the corner. It thus may replace the gold standard. When the method does no better than randomly assigning, the points lie around a straight line (dotted line, fig. 2). Accordingly, the area under the ROC curve can be used as a measure of quality of discrimination, a very 'good' method giving a value 1, and a 'useless' method giving 0.5. Another example of a ROC curve for the same method has been constructed by Ricketts et al. [9].

We have pointed out earlier that the method of validation depends on the intended use of the method. This translates in this category of validations to the statement that the choice of the most preferable cutoff depends on the application. Not in all applications is the point of the curve closest to the upper left corner the 'best' point, corresponding to the 'best' cutoff value. In an application in which the user wants a high sensitivity and does not care much about the specificity (a treatment-eager diagnostician), a low cutoff will be chosen. A user of the ECM that wants to be certain that no sound fissures are treated chooses a high cutoff. However, when there is no preference to achieve either a high specificity or high sensitivity at the cost of severely deteriorating the other, then the contact point between the ROC curve and its tangent under 45° gives the preferable cutoff (fig. 2).

Validation by Comparison with a Method that Is Known Not to Be a Gold Standard

More often than not, methods are validated against a secondary standard. This, in turn, is once or more often calibrated against the true standard. Then the following question comes up: suppose the relation between standard and secondary standard is known, and the relation between the new method and secondary standard is measured, what is the relation between the new method and true standard? Two cases will be considered: all three methods produce continuous parameters which are linearly related, and all three methods are dichotomous.

When all three methods produce a continuous parameter and are linearly related, the question reduces to the calculation of a correlation coefficient

$r_{\text{new-standard}}$ ($r_{\text{n-st}}$) from the coefficients $r_{\text{secondary standard - standard}}$ ($r_{\text{ss-st}}$) and $r_{\text{new-secondary standard}}$ ($r_{\text{n-ss}}$), and construction of the regression line of 'new' on 'standard'.

For the correlation coefficient $r_{\text{n-st}}$ only a lower and an upper limit can be calculated. Using the formula for the partial correlation coefficient [10] and inserting its limits ± 1, one can find limits for $r_{\text{n-st}}$:

$$\text{Limits } (r_{\text{n-st}}) = r_{\text{n-ss}} \times r_{\text{ss-st}} \pm \sqrt{[r_{\text{n-ss}} \times r_{\text{ss-st}})^2 - (r_{\text{n-ss}})^2 - (r_{\text{ss-st}})^2 + 1]},$$

the plus and minus signs refer to the maximum and minimum value of $r_{\text{n-st}}$, respectively. Of course, $r_{\text{n-st}}$ is also limited by the general limit: $r_{\text{n-st}} \leq 1$. This upper boundary can only be reached in our field by unusually high values of $r_{\text{n-ss}}$ and $r_{\text{ss-st}}$.

The case that all three methods are dichotomous was considered by Verdonschot et al. [11]. These authors considered validation of fiber-optic transillumination for approximal caries against bitewing radiography and histology as secondary and primary standards, respectively. Their derivation requires a crucial assumption: namely that the distribution between *truly* sound and *truly* diseased objects is the same in both the group diagnosed by the new method as diseased and the group diagnosed by the new method as sound. This assumption is not explicitly stated in their paper, although their discussion indicates that they are aware of it. Unfortunately, it is very unlikely that this assumption is justified. Therefore we propose that this method only be applied when this assumption has been checked thoroughly.

Another problem with indirect validation of dichotomous methods is that the specificity and sensitivity of the secondary standard versus the true standard have to be taken from the literature. However, as pointed out in an earlier section, these quantities depend upon the composition of the sample, i.e. the method by which the sample was taken from the population and of the properties of the population itself. Thus it should be checked whether or not the literature values pertain to a similar sample as the sample under consideration. Verdonschot et al. [11] discuss this point for the case investigated by them.

We conclude that for any type of quantity, the use of a secondary standard is very inferior to the use of the established gold standard. Secondary standards should be avoided whenever possible.

Validation of a Method that Is Expected to Be 'Better' than the Present Gold Standard

Progress in diagnostic science means that new methods are better than existing ones, including the agreed 'gold standard' of that moment. This conflicts with the notion that any new method should be validated against the present gold standard. This conflict has to be solved by reasoning and the weighing of arguments rather than by following a prescription. This corresponds to our statement in an earlier section that a gold standard is a matter of choice by the investigator of the method or by protocolled agreement of diagnosticians. At least the following arguments should play a role when the replacement of a gold standard is considered: reproducibility, amount and quality of information provided, validity in the sense of relation to diagnostic aim. Preferably but not forcibly, research should be done to support the arguments.

When the reproducibility of a new method is better, i.e. shows a lower standard deviation, than that of existing methods, then it is probably preferable provided the validity is the same or better. An example of such a discussion is given by Clark et al. [12] in their table 2. When the amount and quality of information provided by a new method is better than by existing methods, the diagnostician will make a better decision and thus the new method is preferable, provided of course that the information is relevant for the aim of the diagnosis. Thus, e.g., a quantitative method will be preferable over a dichotomous method. The ECM, cited above, is an example. Or, a method that provides an image and a number will be preferable over a method that provides an image or a number only. The quantitative light-induced fluorescence method for incipient caries lesions is an example [13]. Lastly, a method that enables nondestructive time-dependent monitoring of one and the same specimen is another example of increase of information. Replacement of destructive methods, like microhardness and histology, with non-destructive methods is common in caries research [14–16]. Validation then should be done against the final situation, determined either clinically or by histology [16].

When a new method relates closer to the intended use than the presently available ones, the new one is preferable, provided the reproducibility and amount of information are at least as good as that of existing methods. The periodontal probe developed by Jeffcoat et al. [17] is an example. It determines pocket depth from the cemento-enamel junction, which better corresponds to the clinically relevant attachment loss than the traditional probes. These measure from the edge of the gingiva, which as well may have retracted in the process of attachment loss.

Often research on the validity will have to use destructive methods. For instance, determination of pocket depth with the new pocket probe [17] was validated in a beagle dog model against the diagnostically more relevant quantity 'true attachment', determined after extraction of the tooth. The use of magnetic resonance imaging to determine disc displacement as a component of the diagnosis of temporomandibular joint disorders was validated on cadaver material against histology [18]. Methods to determine the momentary status of caries lesions should, by consensus of involved researchers, be compared with the mineral content of the lesion as determined by transverse microradiography of lesion slices as a gold standard [19]. This does not imply, though, that mineral content is the quantity most relevant for caries activity in that lesion.

Destructive methods have the important disadvantage that they can only be repeated on the destroyed object (extracted, sliced, cut, etc.), but not on the original object of measurement. It then has to be made certain that the location measured with either or both methods is the most relevant one, or that both methods measure the same, respectively. This requires special precautions, such as markings.

Conclusions

In summary then: (1) diagnosis involves the determination of disease and disease activity, of which determination of signs and symptoms is only a part; (2) repeatability, reproducibility, accuracy and validity are distinguishable and well-defined quantities to characterize a new method; (3) quantitative methods should not be reduced to qualitative ones by the use of a cutoff, rather the diagnostician should use all available information; (4) a new method should be characterized by comparison with the current gold standard, the use of a secondary standard is very inferior; (5) sensitivity and specificity are preferably determined in a randomly selected sample, when this is impossible the method of sampling and the composition of the sample should be given, and (6) the choice of a gold standard is a matter of reasoning and weighing of conflicting arguments rather than of following a procedure.

Acknowledgements

We thank Karin Trollsås (Huddinge) and Marie-Charlotte Huysmans (Groningen) for digging up the original data that were used to construct figures 1 and 2, respectively.

References

1 Proceedings of a conference on diagnostic and therapeutic technology in dentistry. Adv Dent Res 1987;1:1–132.
2 Modern concepts in the diagnosis of oral disease. Proc 12th Int Conf Oral Biol, Edinburgh, 1992. Adv Dent Res 1993;7:62–240.
3 Stookey GK (ed): Early Detection of Dental Caries. Indianapolis, Indiana University, 1996.

4 Verdonschot EH, Angmar-Månsson B, ten Bosch JJ, Deery Ch, Huysmans MCDNJM, Pitts NB, Waller E: Developments in caries diagnosis and their relationship to treatment decisions and quality of care. ORCA Afternoon Symposium 1997. Caries Res 1999;33:32–40.
5 Jeffcoat MK, Reddy MS: Advances in measurements of periodontal bone and attachment loss; in Faller RV (ed): Assessment of Oral Health: Diagnostic Techniques and Validation Criteria. Monogr Oral Sci. Basel, Karger, 2000, vol 17, pp 56–72.
6 Biesbrock A, Yeh CH: Relationship of surface epithelium concentrations of IL-1α and IL-1β to clinical inflammation during experimental gingivitis; in Faller RV (ed): Assessment of Oral Health: Diagnostic Techniques and Validation Criteria. Monogr Oral Sci. Basel, Karger, 2000, vol 17, pp 20–31.
7 Lussi A: Impact of including or excluding cavitated lesions when evaluating methods for the diagnosis of occlusal caries. Caries Res 1996;30:389–393.
8 Huysmans MCDNJM, Longbottom C, Pitts NB: Electrical methods in occlusal caries diagnosis: An in-vitro comparison with visual inspection and bite-wing radiography. Caries Res 1998;32: 324–329.
9 Ricketts DNJ, Kidd EAM, Liepins PJ, Wilson RF: Histological validation of electrical resistance measurements in the diagnosis of occlusal caries. Caries Res 1996;30:148–155.
10 Pedhazur EJ: Multiple Regression in Behavioral Research. Explanation and Reduction, ed 2. New York, Holt, Rinehart & Winston, 1982, p 103.
11 Verdonschot EH, Bronkhorst EM, Wenzel A: Approximal caries diagnosis using fiber-optic transillumination: A mathematical adjustment to improve validity. Community Dent Oral Epidemiol 1991; 19:329–332.
12 Clark GT, Delcanho RE, Goulet J-P: The utility and validity of current diagnostic procedures for defining temporomandibular disorder patients. Adv Dent Res 1993;7:97–112.
13 Angmar-Månsson B, Al-Khateeb S, Tranaeus S: Intraoral use of quantitative light-induced fluorescence for caries detection; in Stookey GK (ed): Early Detection of Dental Caries. Indianapolis, Indiana University, 1996, pp 105–118.
14 Al-Khateeb S, Oliveby A, de Josselin de Jong E, Angmar-Månsson B: Laser fluorescence quantification of remineralisation in situ of incipient enamel lesions: Influence of fluoride supplements. Caries Res 1997;31:132–140.
15 Øgaard B, ten Bosch JJ: Regression of white spot enamel lesions. A new optical method for quantitative longitudinal evaluation in vivo. Am J Orthod Dent Orthop 1993;8:238–242.
16 Anderson P, Davis GR, Ahluwahlia MHK: Monitoring de- and remineralisation of enamel in vitro using an infrared reflectance meter. Caries Res 1996;30:394–399.
17 Jeffcoat MK, Jeffcoat RL, Captain K: A periodontal probe with automated cemento-enamel junction detection – Design and clinical trials. IEEE Trans Biomed Eng 1991;38:330–334.
18 Westesson P-L: Reliability and validity of imaging diagnosis of temporomandibular joint disorders. Adv Dent Res 1993;7:137–151.
19 Featherstone JDB: Consensus conference on intra-oral models: Evaluation techniques. J Dent Res 1992;71(special issue):955–956.

Prof. Jaap J. ten Bosch, Department Biomedical Engineering, University of Groningen,
Ant. Deusinglaan 1, 9713 AV Groningen (The Netherlands)
Tel. +31 50 3633138, Fax +31 50 3633159, E-Mail J.J.ten.Bosch@med.rug.nl

Author Index

Subject Index